THE

Good Morning

MACROBIOTIC

Breakfast Book

THE
Good Morning
MACROBIOTIC
Breakfast Book

AVELINE KUSHI
WENDY ESKO

FOREWORD BY WILLIAM P. CASTELLI, MD

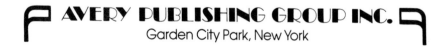
AVERY PUBLISHING GROUP INC.
Garden City Park, New York

Cover Design: Janine Eisner-Wall and Rudy Shur
Front Cover Photograph Credit: SuperStock, Inc.
In-House Editor: Marie Caratozzolo
Typesetter: Pro-To-Type Unlimited

Library of Congress Cataloging-in-Publication Data

Kushi, Aveline.
  The good morning macrobiotic breakfast book / Aveline Kushi, Wendy
Esko.
    p. cm.
  Includes bibliographical references and index.
  ISBN 0-89529-442-7
  1. Breakfasts. 2. Cookery (Natural foods) I. Esko, Wendy.
  II. Title.
  TX733.K87 1991   90-14441
                                                        CIP

Printed in the United States of America

10 9 8 7 6 5 4 3 2

Contents

Preface

One the first questions people ask when they hear the word macrobiotics is, "What do you eat for breakfast?" Although the tradition of eating oatmeal, corn grits, buckwheat pancakes, and other cereal grains in the morning goes back hundreds of years, for someone accustomed to starting the day with a meal of bacon and eggs or coffee and donuts, the notion of having hot cereal, soup, vegetables, and tofu as breakfast fare may sound new and exotic. You will discover in the pages of this book that the foods included in the macrobiotic diet have been the mainstay of healthful diets for centuries, and can easily be adapted by contemporary cooks to create a wide variety of nourishing and delicious breakfast dishes.

Today's modern breakfast is very high in cholesterol, saturated fat, sugar, chemical additives, and refined foods. For many people, breakfast is the most hazardous meal of the day. Fortunately, the macrobiotic diet can help everyone avoid these potential hazards and begin each day healthfully. The foods included most often in macrobiotic breakfasts are cholesterol-free and very low in saturated fat. They contain no refined sugar, are high in complex carbohydrates and fiber, and meet the nutritional guidelines set by leading public health agencies. Macrobiotic breakfasts are also simple and fun to prepare.

For readers new to macrobiotics, we include a description of the wide range of foods included in the standard macrobiotic diet, and present guidelines for using these foods at breakfast. We also discuss the preliminary steps involved in macrobiotic cooking, including the selection of high-quality foods and utensils, and the basic guidelines for washing and cutting foods properly. The recipes offered generally follow the order of the standard macrobiotic diet—beginning with a variety of whole grain porridges and other grain dishes, and followed by suggestions for preparing morning miso and other soups, fresh vegetable dishes, tofu and soy-product dishes, condiments, and caffeine-free beverages. In the final chapter, we present a variety of "special occasion" breakfast dishes, ranging from whole grain waffles and pancakes with natural toppings, to scrambled tofu, whole wheat donuts, and cinnamon-raisin rolls.

We wish to thank everyone who contributed to *The Good Morning Macrobiotic Breakfast Book*. We thank Dr. William Castelli, director of the Framingham Heart Study, for contributing a foreword, and for his continuing effort to enlighten people everywhere about the relationship between diet, cholesterol, and heart disease. We wish to thank Michio Kushi for his untiring dedication to world health and peace, and for furthering the understanding of the macrobiotic approach to diet and health. We also thank Edward Esko for his guidance in writing this book, and Alex Jack for providing background research on the history and nutritional value of the foods included in the recipes. We also thank Rudy Shur, Marie Caratozzolo, and other members of the Avery staff for their guidance and assistance.

Aveline Kushi
Wendy Esko
Becket, Massachusetts

Foreword

It has only been recently that we have been able to look inside the arteries of the necks of people involved in the Framingham Heart Study. Of the men and women over the age of sixty-five, 70 percent have a deposit of cholesterol big enough so that I can see it easily with a machine that uses ultrasound to look non-invasively into the arteries located near the surface of the body. Of these men and women, 10 percent have an artery blockage of 50 percent or more. Once deposits of cholesterol are in these arteries of the neck, it means that they are already in the heart arteries. The disease begins when we are children and starts in the big blood vessel located in the abdomen. It then spreads to the arteries of the heart, then to the arteries in the chest, and then on to the legs. From there, the blockages spread to the neck and eventually to the inside of the head. Every day we tend to lay down another layer of cholesterol, and the older we get, the closer we get to shutting down a critical artery in our body. When we shut down an artery in our heart, we have a heart attack; when we shut down an artery in our head, the result is a stroke. If an artery shuts down in a leg, we could lose part of the leg.

For most of us, this process begins at breakfast when we pile on a ton of fat that includes too much cholesterol and too much of what is called saturated fat. Saturated fat causes the body to manufacture cholesterol, and most of the cholesterol in our bodies is manufactured by our bodies; it does not come from eating cholesterol itself. More than 4 billion of the 5 billion or so people who live on this Earth do not get this disease of cholesterol deposits. This is because they do not eat the kind of breakfasts that most Americans eat. Instead, they eat the kind of breakfasts described in this book. In rural Japan, not only are the people free from these cholesterol deposits, but they have become the people who live to be the oldest.

We have started the cholesterol campaign in America to help you understand how important it is to find out what your cholesterol level is at as early an age as possible. If this cholesterol level becomes elevated, you must start to change it to prevent a heart attack. About half of the people in America die prematurely from these cholesterol deposits; one-third of the men and women in our country have either a heart attack or stroke before the age of sixty-five, and this rate doubles after sixty-five. If your total cholesterol is over 150 mg/dl (milligrams per deciliter of blood) or your triglyceride level is over 150 mg/dl, it is important for you to have enough of a kind of cholesterol in your blood called the high-density lipoprotein (HDL) cholesterol to protect you. The simplest way to establish this is to divide your total cholesterol by your HDL cholesterol. If the number you come up with is 4.5 or higher, you are in a dangerous setting. A ratio under 3.5 is approaching ideal, and between these numbers, we think your deposits of cholesterol are growing, but at such a slow rate that you will probably have to make it to an old age before having a heart attack.

There are no magic bullets! You must start to look critically at your life and introduce changes if necessary. By making changes in diet and exercise, and stopping bad habits like smoking, you will be giving your body the best chance possible to stay healthy for as long as possible. In diet, it means finding as few as six or seven recipes that you enjoy eating. You won't continue to eat something you don't like for the rest of your life, even if you know it will save your life. The importance of this book is that it offers a large variety of recipes that should appeal to people with many different tastes. Keep trying different recipes; don't be discouraged if you try a recipe you don't like. Eventually, you should find enough recipes so that you can look forward to breakfasts you enjoy eating, and at the same time, not adding to those cholesterol deposits. The greatest news is that the deposits are reversible; the diets in this book will be a big step toward starting the reversibility process in your body. Your arteries could actually be better one year from now instead of being worse.

As my French friends say: Bon Appetit!

William P. Castelli, MD
Framingham, Massachusetts

Chapter One
START THE DAY RIGHT

The Earth turns. A faint glimmer of light in the east heralds the beginning of a new day. Soon the sun will rise over the horizon, bringing with it light and warmth. The mist on the mountains will vanish, as will the cool, moist dew in the gardens. Everywhere people stir and become active. A new day has started. It is time to break the night's fast. It is time for breakfast!

During sleep we re-energize ourselves. As the Earth turns away from the sun toward the outer reaches of space at night, a countless number of stars shower the planet with light and energy. By not eating at night, we make ourselves more sensitive to these vibrations. It is not until the following morning that we break our fast. The foods we eat in the morning influence how we think and feel during the rest of the day. Breakfast is a very important meal.

THE DAILY CYCLE

Health comes from living in harmony with nature. Understanding the cycles of nature makes it easier for us to orient our lives in accord with the environment. As we know from daily experience with the weather, the atmosphere is constantly changing. In the morning, light, heat, and solar radiation charge and enliven the planet. All things on Earth react to this strong charge of energy. Flowers that close their petals at night open as soon as they are touched by the sun's rays. Similarly, we open our eyes, stretch, and get up in the morning. Morning is a time of actively rising and newly erupting energy, similar to that of spring. Evening has an opposite quality. It is a time of quiet, downward energy, similar to that of autumn and winter.

Day to day and season to season, the movements of nature cycle back and forth between expansion and contraction, or *yin* and *yang*. The movement of water offers a good example. The expanding phase of the cycle begins when water evaporates and rises into the atmosphere. This upward movement peaks high above the earth when clouds appear. Then it condenses into droplets and falls back to earth. This gathering or contracting part of the cycle becomes stronger as water collects in rivers, streams, lakes, and, ultimately, in the ocean. When temperatures are cold enough, water condenses into crystals of ice. When ice melts in the spring, the cycle starts over again.

Our daily routine is also governed by expanding and contracting movement. The rising energy of morning compels us to exchange the horizontal position of sleep for a vertical standing position. It also activates us physically and mentally, to the extent that many of us leave the house and venture out into the world. Outward movement reaches a peak around noon, at which time we pause to eat lunch. Atmospheric energy changes direction in the afternoon and starts to move downward, at which time we tend to become quiet and reflective. The downward movement of the atmosphere becomes most pronounced around sunset, at which time we return home. Evening is often a time of quiet relaxation, and the strong charge of downward energy eventually compels us to lie down and sleep. As the sun rises, the cycle begins again.

Applying our understanding of the daily cycle of energy is a key to health and longevity. The aim of macrobiotic cooking is to prepare meals that help align our body and mind with the flow of energy in the environment. In order to apply this understanding to our cooking, we must first see how to classify daily foods in terms of their energy qualities.

CLASSIFYING FOODS

All foods can be classified according to whether they accelerate expanding or contracting energy. Certain foods are extremely contracting. They contain an abundance of hard, saturated fat and cholesterol, and when eaten in excess, cause hardening and stagnation throughout the body. For the most part, animal foods can be classified in this category. Animals represent the condensation of a great deal of plant foods. We think of foods such as meat, eggs, hard cheese, chicken, shellfish, and red meat or blue-skinned fish as extreme forms of very condensed energy.

Pesticides and the Food Chain

As we move up the food chain from plants to animals, yang, or contracting energy, becomes stronger. This causes the toxic chemicals
used in agriculture to accumulate in animal tissues to a far greater
degree than they do in plants. According to John Robbins, author of
Diet for a New America, 95 to 99 percent of all pesticides and other
toxic residues in the American diet come from meat, dairy products,
eggs, and other animal foods. On the other hand, plant foods contain relatively low concentrations of chemical residues. We can sub-
stantially reduce our intake of these substances by eating whole
grains, beans, fresh local vegetables, and other foods that are lower
on the food chain, and by selecting organically grown foods whenever possible.

On the other hand, certain other foods have an opposite quality. We
can think of them as being strongly charged with extremely expansive
energy. Simple sugars, such as those in refined sugar, honey, and tropical
fruits, offer a good example. Simple sugars are made up of simple glucose molecules that exist either alone (monosaccharides) or in pairs (di-
saccharides). Like the molecules of a gas or liquid, they are not bound
together and have the tendency to rapidly diffuse. They are quickly
absorbed into the bloodstream and produce a short-lived burst of energy
that is followed by a rapid low. The net result of eating them is a gradual
depletion of our health and vitality. Spices are also charged with strong
expanding energy. When we eat them, the capillaries near the surface of
our bodies expand and we become flushed or feel warm. A similar reac-
tion occurs with alcohol, which is also an extremely yin, or expansive,
substance.

Drugs and medications have extremely expansive effects. Synthetic
estrogen, or DES (diethylstilbestrol), offers a good example. This highly
potent substance has been used since World War II to fatten and speed
the growth of livestock. When people eat foods that contain residues of
DES, a variety of biochemical imbalances are set in motion, including the
abnormal development of female sexual characteristics, such as the
growth of breasts in men and young children. Minute dosages can also
trigger the explosive growth of cells known as cancer. Aspirin, which
thins the blood and causes capillaries to expand, is also an extremely yin
product, as are antibiotics, such as those fed to livestock to fatten them
for market.

Complex carbohydrates, or polysaccharides, such as those in whole grains, beans, vegetables, and sea vegetables, are made up of many molecules of glucose linked together in long chains. They are held together by a strong (although not extreme) contracting force. They exist in their natural state along with minerals, proteins, vitamins, and fiber as part of nutritionally balanced whole foods. They are not absorbed as rapidly as simple sugars; instead, they produce a slow, steady release of energy that helps in maintaining an even level of glucose in the blood. Simple sugars produce rapid fluctuations in blood glucose. Because of their simpler, more primitive structures, they can be thought of as fragmented or decomposed forms of complex carbohydrates.

Complex carbohydrates are centrally balanced in terms of yin and yang, or expansive and contractive energies. They have been the mainstay of traditional diets for centuries and are also the primary foods in the macrobiotic diet. Leading public health agencies have started to recognize their value and have suggested that people eat more of them in order to reduce the risk of heart disease, certain cancers, obesity, and other chronic illnesses.

In Table 1.1 foods are classified according to their energy qualities. Strong yang or contractive foods are listed in the column on the left, centrally balanced foods in the center, and the more expansive foods in the column on the right. In general, whole cereal grains are at the center of the food spectrum. They contain an optimal balance of minerals, proteins, carbohydrates, vitamins, and fiber, and are well suited for human dietary needs. The majority of our teeth—the molars and premolars—are perfectly suited for crushing and grinding whole grains, beans, seeds, and other plant fibers. Of course, wide variations in the degree of expanding and contracting energy exist within each category. The foods in each column are arranged from the most contractive to the most expansive. Refined salt, for example, is a condensed mineral and is more yang than meat, eggs, or cheese. Beef, pork, and eggs are more condensed than poultry or fish.

Within the centrally balanced column, grains are in the center, and beans, which are usually larger and higher in fat than grains, are more yin or expansive. Vegetables are generally larger and more expansive than grains or beans; while fruits, oils, and concentrated sweeteners, such as rice syrup and barley malt, are generally the most expansive foods in the centrally balanced category.

Among extremely yin foods, refined grains, tropical fruits, nightshade vegetables, and refined oils, although very extreme, are less expansive than refined sugar, chemicals, drugs, and medications. In general, an optimal diet is based around complex carbohydrates and other foods in

Table 1.1 General Yin (∇) and Yang (Δ) Classification of Food

Strong Yang Foods	More Balanced Foods	Strong Yin Foods
Refined salt	Unrefined white sea salt,	White rice, white flour
Eggs	miso, tamari soy sauce,	Frozen and canned foods
Meat	and other naturally salty	Tropical fruits and vegeta-
Hard cheese	seasonings	bles including those orig-
Poultry	Tekka, gomashio, umeboshi,	inating in the tropics—
Lobster, crab, and other	and other naturally pro-	e.g., tomatoes and pota-
shellfish	cessed salty condiments	toes
Red meat and blue-skinned	Low-fat, white-meat fish	Milk, cream, yogurt, and
fish	Sea vegetables	ice cream
	Whole cereal grains	Refined oils
	Beans and bean products	Spices (pepper, curry, nut-
	Root, round, and leafy green	meg, etc.)
	vegetables from temper-	Aromatic and stimulant
	ate climates	beverages (coffee, black
	Fruits grown in temperate	tea, mint tea, etc.)
	climates	Honey, sugar, and refined
	Nonaromatic, nonstimu-	sweeteners
	lant beverages	Alcohol
	Spring or well water	Foods containing chemi-
	Naturally processed veg-	cals, preservatives, dyes,
	etable oils	and pesticides
	Brown rice syrup, barley	Artificial sweeteners
	malt, and other natural	Drugs (marijuana, cocaine,
	grain-based sweeteners	etc., with a few excep-
	(when used moderately)	tions)
		Medications (tranquilizers,
		antibiotics, etc., with some
		exceptions)

Source: *The Macrobiotic Cancer Prevention Cookbook*, Aveline Kushi and Wendy Esko (Avery Publishing Group, 1988).

the centrally balanced category, and minimizes or avoids the use of extremely expansive or contractive items.

There is also a tremendous range of variation within each type of food. For example, among the grains and their immediate relatives, buckwheat, millet, and winter wheat are more contracted, while summer wheat, barley, and corn contain more expanding energies. Brown rice is generally in between, but again, this depends on the variety being considered. Short grain rice, which is the most suitable variety for temperate climates, is generally the most balanced, while the medium and long grain varieties, used in warmer regions, are more expansive. Similarly, larger beans, which are higher in fat, are more yin than smaller, low-fat varieties. Dense, compact root vegetables are more contracting than expanded leafy greens. Vegetables and fruits that originate in warm tropical climates are, for the most part, more yin than varieties that come from temperate or cold climates. In order to maintain optimal health in a temperate zone, it is better to minimize or avoid the intake of fruits, vegetables, spices, coffee, sugar, chocolate, and other foods that come from the tropics.

EATING WITH THE DAILY CYCLE

Many of you may be familiar with our book *The Changing Seasons Macrobiotic Cookbook* (Avery, 1985). In it we present a wide range of menus and a variety of recipes that can help you adjust your cooking according to the seasonal cycle. By emphasizing certain energies in our dishes at different times of the year, we are better able to harmonize the condition of our bodies with the changing atmosphere.

Adjustments such as these are subtle and require sensitivity to the energy around us. They are also made within the context of the standard macrobiotic diet, which is based on the use of centrally balanced foods. Seasonal adjustments in diet are also flexible and dynamic. We need plenty of variety in our diets throughout the year, and need to prepare a wide variety of dishes in each season. So, for example, although we recommend emphasizing the contractive energies in foods during autumn and winter, we still need plenty of fresh leafy greens in order to avoid becoming one-sided in our cooking and eating. We also need strongly cooked dishes during the spring and summer, when our cooking tends to become lighter, in order to maintain strength and vitality. As you can see, variety and flexibility are key ingredients in adapting these guidelines successfully. The same principle applies to cooking in harmony with the daily cycle.

As we have seen, morning is a time when light, rising energy predominates in the atmosphere. If we wish to be harmonious with this energy, breakfast is best kept light and simple. Foods such as eggs, cheese, bacon, sausage, and ham are very contracting. Eating them for breakfast blocks the natural upward movement of energy in the morning. This leads to feelings of heaviness or stagnation that make it more difficult to be physically and mentally alert during the day. It is far better to base our breakfast on vegetable-quality foods that contain more light, expansive energy.

Eating less in the morning is also better for health and vitality. The foods we eat move in a downward direction through the digestive tract. If we eat a large volume of food, this downward motion creates opposition to the upward flow of energy in the morning. A condition of resistance is created that can result in a "stuck" feeling, or can cause difficulty in pursuing the day's activities, or can prevent us from thinking with maximum vitality and clarity. In some cases, especially if a person is overweight, it may be a good idea to eat a very light breakfast or even skip breakfast from time to time, perhaps having only tea or another beverage in the morning. Another way to prevent eating too much at breakfast (or at any other meal) is to chew each mouthful thoroughly. When you chew whole grains, vegetables, and other complex-carbohydrate foods, they become more digestible and release rich, naturally sweet flavors. We recommend chewing each mouthful thirty to fifty times.

Eating too much, or basing breakfast on calorically dense foods, such as meat, eggs, or cheese, creates disharmony with the environment. Whole grains, vegetables, and other centrally balanced, vegetable-quality foods do not block the smooth flow of energy. By making simple adjustments in the way we cook breakfast foods, we can fine tune the alignment of energy in our dishes.

In general, breakfast foods should be softer and easier to digest than the dishes served at other meals. For example, breakfast grains are generally cooked with more water than the grain dishes served at lunch or dinner. Additional water makes the grains softer and more expanded, thus harmonizing their energy with that of the morning. For this reason, soft porridges made with whole grains are usually the main dishes in macrobiotic breakfasts. Vegetable side dishes are also cooked in ways that accelerate light, expansive energy. Quick steaming, boiling, and quick sautéing activate upward energy. These preparation methods are often used in macrobiotic breakfasts. Natural fermentation is also a more expansive process and matches the light, upward energy of morning. Naturally fermented foods, such as miso and quickly fermented pickles, can also be served at breakfast. Miso made with fermented barley (a light expansive grain) is especially good when used to make morning miso soup. Simple adjustments such as these are the keys to eating for good health.

A CHOLESTEROL-FREE BREAKFAST

Aside from being unbalanced in terms of energy, there is another problem with modern breakfast foods—they are often incredibly high in cholesterol and saturated fat. A typical high-fat breakfast may also contain a hefty dose of pesticides or other chemicals due to the concentration of toxic residues in the fat cells of animals.

The relationship between a diet high in fat and cholesterol with heart disease and certain cancers is now widely recognized. Large-scale population studies have revealed that people who consume less cholesterol and saturated fat have lower levels of blood cholesterol and a lower incidence of heart disease. Conversely, people who eat large amounts of saturated fat and cholesterol have higher blood cholesterols and a greater incidence of heart disease. Similar correlations have been found between fat consumption and certain cancers, especially cancers of the colon, breast, and prostate.

However, despite repeated warning about the dangers of eating too much fat and cholesterol, Americans still consume about 37 percent of their calories as fat, with about 13 percent coming from saturated fat. The average daily cholesterol intake for men is 435 milligrams, while 304 milligrams is the average for women. Most experts, including those in the United States Government, agree that this is too much. In February 1990, the government announced a campaign to get virtually the entire nation to eat no more than 10 percent of its calories as saturated fat and no more than 30 percent as total fat, and to take in fewer than 300 milligrams of cholesterol each day. These recommendations, which are supported by thirty-eight private medical and public health organizations, are at the core of a new national campaign to reduce the average American's cholesterol level by 10 percent.

The average person in the United States today has a blood cholesterol level of 225 mg/dl (milligrams of cholesterol per deciliter of blood). Many have levels that are far higher. However, most researchers feel that this average is too high, since the risk of heart attack increases dramatically as cholesterol levels go beyond the range of 160 to 180 mg/dl. As we can see, many people have cholesterol levels that put them at risk for heart attacks and other cardiovascular disorders. Dr. William Castelli, director of the Framingham Heart Study, reported that the risk of heart attack virtually disappears in persons with cholesterol levels below 150 mg/dl. These are the levels found in people who use very little animal food in their diets. Eating a naturally balanced diet could be the best way to lower your blood cholesterol and your risk of heart disease.

Recent studies have also shown that diet alone can actually reverse blockages in the arteries, the chief cause of heart attacks and strokes in the United States. In November 1989, a study was released by cardiologist Dean Ornish and his colleagues at the University of California at San Francisco. In this study, forty-eight volunteers ate a very low-fat, primarily vegetarian diet that excluded poultry, high-fat dairy products, red meat, oils, and fats. Through this diet alone, the volunteers were able to partially clear their blocked arteries. Claude J. M. Lenfant, director of the National Heart, Lung, and Blood Institute, said the most interesting aspect of the study was the finding that changes in diet and lifestyle alone "can be just as effective in reversing blocked arteries as cholesterol-lowering drugs."

Aside from preventing heart disease, a balanced diet may also offer a natural, drug-free way to reverse already existing circulatory blockages. Dr. William Castelli, in *Lessons From the Framingham Heart Study, Cancer and Heart Disease: the Macrobiotic Approach* (Japan Publications, 1982), states:

> *Diet is related in a very important way to the level of our blood cholesterols. Animal meats contain mostly cholesterol and saturated fat; two kinds of fat which elevate our bad cholesterols—particularly LDL [low density lipoprotein] cholesterol—which many feel is the major cholesterol deposited in our blood vessel walls. Polyunsatu-*

rated fat, which is found in vegetable oils like corn oil, safflower oil, sunflower seed oil, and others, lowers the bad cholesterols in our blood. Egg yolks rich in cholesterol are to be avoided. Dairy fat is likewise dangerous, because it raises the bad cholesterols…Some people say that because our body manufactures cholesterol it does not matter what we eat, but this is totally false. People who eat little saturated fat or cholesterols have cholesterols so low in this country that they virtually appear to be immune to this disease [heart disease]. When the body does not get very much saturated fat or cholesterol in the diet, our cholesterols average about 125 mg. percent [mg/dl] instead of the usual 225 mg. percent [mg/dl] found in Framingham.

In Table 1.2, the cholesterol and fat content of some common breakfast foods are presented. As you can see, most are quite high in total fat,

Table 1.2   Cholesterol and Fat Content of Modern Breakfast Foods

Food	Portion	Cholesterol (mg)	Total Fat (gm)	Saturated Fat (gm)
Fast-food ham and cheese omelet	1 serving	525	19	—
Fast-food scrambled eggs	1 serving	514	13	5
Fast-food sausage and egg biscuit	1	285	40	15
Fast-food egg muffin	1	259	16	6
French toast	1 slice	112	7	2
Cream cheese	3 ounces	93	30	19
Cheese danish	1	48	22	6
Egg bagel	1	44	2	trace
Corn muffin (from mix)	1.6 ounces	42	6	2
Fast-food pork sausage	1 serving	39	19	7
Whole milk	1 cup	35	9	6
Butter	1 tablespoon	30	11	7
American cheese	1 ounce	25	8	5
Glazed donut	2.1 ounces	21	13	5
Bacon	3 medium slices	16	9	3
English muffin with butter	1	15	5	2
Hash brown potatoes	1 serving	7	9	4

Source: *Food Values: Cholesterol and Fats* by Leah Wallach. Copyright 1989 by Harper & Row, Publishers, Inc. Reprinted by permission of HarperCollins Publishers.

saturated fat, and cholesterol. A breakfast based on these foods can push a person's daily cholesterol intake far beyond the United States Government's Recommended Daily Allowance. Suppose, for example, someone stops off at a fast-food restaurant on the way to work and orders scrambled eggs, a corn muffin with two pats of butter, hash brown potatoes, an order of pork sausage, and a glass of milk. Let's see what the cholesterol count is for this one meal, based on the figures given in Table 1.2.

Food	Cholesterol
Scrambled eggs	514
Pork sausage	39
Corn muffin	42
Butter	30
Hash browns	7
Glass of milk	35
Total cholesterol	667

The cholesterol count for this meal alone is 667 milligrams. That is *more than double* the government's daily recommended allowance! Moreover, according to the amounts given in Table 1.2, this modern breakfast adds 67 grams of total fat and 31 grams of saturated fat to the diet. Clearly, the modern breakfast puts many people at greater risk of heart disease.

Now let's compare these figures with those of the macrobiotic diet. In terms of overall balance, about 15 percent of the calories in a macrobiotic diet come from fat, with about 2 percent being saturated. Both of these amounts are safely below the government's suggested allowance. It is important to remember that the macrobiotic diet is based primarily on plant foods, which contain no cholesterol and very little saturated fat. In Table 1.3, the cholesterol and fat content of the typical natural foods included in macrobiotic breakfasts is presented. They contain no cholesterol and are very low in saturated fat.

Studies conducted on members of the macrobiotic community confirm that eating foods such as these, results in lower cholesterol levels. The average blood cholesterols among people eating macrobiotically is about 125 mg/dl. This was discovered in the mid-1970s by researchers at Harvard Medical School and the Framingham Heart Study. In a study published in the *New England Journal of Medicine*, 116 macrobiotic volunteers, living in the Boston area, were compared with a randomly selected control group consuming the usual American diet. They were matched with the study group by age and sex. The results are summarized as follows:

- Cholesterol levels in the macrobiotic group were found to be strikingly lower than those in the controls and the usual United States levels.

Table 1.3   Cholesterol and Fat Content of Macrobiotic Breakfast Foods

Food	Portion	Cholesterol (mg)	Total Fat (gm)	Saturated Fat (gm)
Brown Rice	1 cup	0	1	trace
Barley	1 cup	0	2	trace
Oat flakes	2 ounces	0	4	trace
Brown rice crispies	1 cup	0	1	trace
Whole wheat flour	1 cup	0	2	trace
Buckwheat flour	1 cup	0	1	trace
Cornmeal	1 cup	0	4	1
Miso	1/2 cup	0	8	1
Tempeh	1/2 cup	0	6	1
Tofu	1/2 cup	0	6	1
Butternut squash	1/2 cup	0	trace	trace
Chinese cabbage	1/2 cup	0	trace	trace
Daikon (Oriental radish)	1/2 cup	0	trace	trace
Onions	1 tablespoon	0	trace	trace
Scallions	1 tablespoon	0	trace	trace
Shiitake (dried Japanese mushrooms)	0.1 ounce	0	trace	trace
Turnip greens	1/2 cup	0	trace	trace
Sesame oil	1 tablespoon	0	14	2
Corn oil	1 tablespoon	0	14	2

Source: *Food Values: Cholesterol and Fats* by Leah Wallach. Copyright 1989 by Harper & Row, Publishers, Inc. Reprinted by permission of HarperCollins Publishers.

- These low levels were found in all age groups. The rise of cholesterol with age, usually significantly steep, was very slight.
- The macrobiotic subjects were also found to weigh less than average. (Obesity is a known risk factor in cardiovascular disease, cancer, diabetes, liver disease, and other chronic illnesses.)
- Animal food consumption appeared to be the major correlating factor in the different cholesterol levels.
- Consumption of dairy products and eggs seemed to have the most direct influence on elevated cholesterol levels.
- The longer the individual had been following the macrobiotic diet, the lower his or her cholesterol level had dropped below the usual levels.

Macrobiotic breakfasts are well within the recommended United States Government allowance for saturated fat and cholesterol. The first meal of the day can be a very good place to start in lowering your daily intake of cholesterol and fat, reducing your risk of heart disease and cancer.

A SUGAR-FREE BREAKFAST

Like the opposite poles of a magnet, yin and yang attract one another. The more extreme the diet becomes at one end, the more we require opposite extremes to create balance. As a result, modern breakfasts, based on high-fat animal foods, often include plenty of sugar, coffee, frozen fruit juices, and other extremely yin foods or beverages.

Today, the average American eats over 100 pounds of sugar per year, much of it at breakfast. Sugar is used as an additive in such common breakfast foods as packaged cereals; fruit jellies; artificially sweetened syrups; pancake, waffle, and muffin mixes; croissants; and sweet rolls. Moreover, people often pour sugar on their hot or cold cereals and add it to morning coffee and tea. Of course, the popular coffee and donut breakfast is based around caffeine and sugar. People also consume simple sugars in the form of frozen orange juice, grapefruit, bananas and other tropical fruits, honey, and maple syrup eaten at breakfast.

However, the intake of refined and other forms of simple sugar, creates imbalances in the body that contribute to ill health. Simple sugars are metabolized quickly and cause the blood to become overacidic. They also produce a rapid rise in blood sugar. To compensate, the pancreas secretes insulin, which causes excess sugar in the blood to be removed and enter the cells of the body. This produces a burst of energy as the glucose, the end product of all sugar metabolism, is oxidized. Once the sugar is metabolized, however, the level of blood sugar often dips below normal, causing a condition known as hypoglycemia. This condition produces the craving for more sugar and sweets, leading to compulsive snacking and unnecessary weight gain. Hypoglycemia also produces symptoms such as fatigue, sleepiness, lack of mental clarity, and depression. These symptoms often become more acute in the late afternoon, when atmospheric energy becomes more downward and still.

Excess sugar is released into the bloodstream as fatty acid and can cause fat to accumulate throughout the body, including in and around the internal organs. The levels of triglycerides (fatty acids) in the blood are elevated by the intake of cane sugar, fruit sugar, dairy sugar, alcohol, and other simple sugars. Elevated triglycerides are associated with a higher risk of heart disease. Sugar also depletes calcium and other minerals, leading to tooth decay and depletion of the bones, as in osteoporosis.

The sweetness in macrobiotic breakfasts comes primarily from the polysaccharide glucose (a form of complex carbohydrate) found in whole grains, beans, and many varieties of vegetables. When chewed properly, these foods release a wonderfully sweet flavor. Additional sweetness is sometimes provided by natural, grain-based sweeteners such as barley malt and rice syrup. These natural products are derived from the complex carbohydrates in whole grains. On occasion, raisins, natural unsweetened jellies, and other sweeteners made from more balanced, temperate fruits can be eaten, but usually in small amounts and as special treats.

OTHER MODERN BREAKFAST DANGERS

The problems with the modern breakfast aren't limited to too much cholesterol, fat, and sugar. Many processed breakfast foods are also high in sodium, while eggs and other animal proteins are usually eaten with plenty of salt. The salt that most people shake on their scrambled eggs is usually refined table salt, a nutritionally deficient product that is almost pure sodium chloride. In macrobiotic cooking, only high-quality natural sea salt, which contains many trace minerals, is used. Sea salt is a more balanced substance; when used in moderate amounts in cooking, it adds important nutrients to our foods.

For many people, the modern breakfast is also very high in refined and processed foods. According to the National Academy of Sciences, about 65 percent of the food consumed in the United States has been refined or processed in some way. Unlike the past, when people would start their day with a bowl of hot porridge made from nourishing whole grains, most of the grains eaten today have been milled and refined. As a result, many of their essential nutrients have been stripped away. So, for most people, the word "cereal" means processed and refined cereals that come in a box, rather than natural, unprocessed whole grains that come from the earth. And because the modern diet is so high in refined foods, many people take vitamin and mineral supplements in order to offset the resulting imbalances and deficiencies. In essence, the vitamins and minerals taken out of whole natural foods are sold back to the consumer in capsule form or are added to devitalized foods in a process known as "enrichment." However, when taken in this unnatural way, vitamins and other nutrients often cause imbalances in the body's overall metabolism. It is far healthier to base one's diet around foods that contain all of the essential nutrients in balanced proportions.

Many breakfast foods also contain chemicals and additives. Artificial fertilizers and toxic herbicides and pesticides are used on the crops that go into breads, cereals, and other foods eaten at breakfast. Today, more than 3,000 additives are used to color, flavor, preserve, and extend the shelf life of foods, including many of those eaten at breakfast. Most commercial livestock and egg-laying hens are fed artificial growth hormones and antibiotics, and their feed is usually contaminated with chemicals. Many of the chemicals found in today's breakfast foods have been linked to a variety of chronic disorders.

Clearly, then, the modern breakfast is not ideal for maintaining optimum health. The macrobiotic breakfast, on the other hand, offers a low-fat, low-cholesterol, additive- and sugar-free alternative. In the chapter that follows we introduce the wide variety of balanced whole foods that make up the macrobiotic diet and that form the basis of a healthful breakfast. Guidelines will also be presented for selecting and preparing foods to harmonize with the daily cycle of energy. The final chapters offer a variety of appetizing and nourishing recipes designed to help you get off to a healthful start each day.

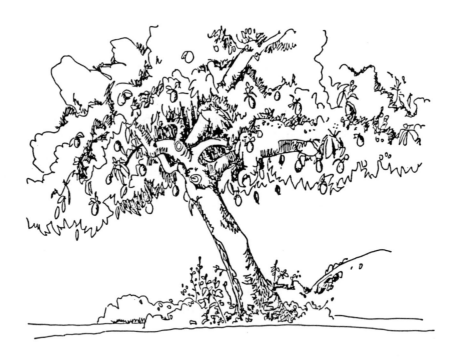

Chapter Two

MACROBIOTIC BREAKFAST FOODS

In this chapter, we introduce the wide range of whole natural foods included in the macrobiotic diet. Even though you probably won't use all of these foods at breakfast, it is a good idea to familiarize yourself with the entire range of healthful foods that can be used in an optimally balanced diet. Thousands of people from around the world have experienced improvements in their health and well-being as the result of adopting this dietary pattern. One of the first benefits that people experience, aside from feeling and looking better, is an immediate drop in their blood cholesterols.

MACROBIOTIC DIETARY GUIDELINES

The standard macrobiotic diet is very much in accord with the latest thinking on preventive health care and nutrition. Preventive guidelines issued by the American Heart Association, the National Academy of Sciences, the U.S. Surgeon General, and other public health agencies recommend a diet high in complex carbohydrates and fiber, and low in fat and cholesterol to reduce the risk of heart disease, cancer, and other chronic illnesses.

The Macrobiotic Nutritional Guidelines (see inset on page 16) are for adults who live in temperate climates. Modifications are necessary if you live in far-northern or tropical zones, or when cooking for babies or children. Of course, each of us has individual dietary needs and preferences, and these must also be considered. Personal guidance is therefore helpful when changing your diet. For this reason we suggest that you attend macrobiotic cooking classes in your area or meet with a qualified macrobiotic advisor. Programs such as the *Macrobiotic Way of Life Seminar* and the *Macrobiotic Residential Seminar*, offered by the Kushi Institute in Massachusetts, are especially recommended. Thousands of people have attended these programs and have found them very useful. A wide variety of books are also available on the nutritional, health, and cooking aspects of macrobiotics. These are listed in the Recommended Reading Section and are suggested for personal study.

The percentages of foods presented below are for an entire day, and are calculated by volume and not by weight. You don't need to include all of these categories at every meal, nor is it necessary to include all of these foods at once, when beginning macrobiotics. You can start with the basic staples and broaden your selection as you familiarize yourself

Macrobiotic Nutritional Guidelines

The nutritional guidelines of macrobiotics are remarkably similar to those included in the United States Government's *Dietary Goals for the United States*, the *Surgeon General's Report on Diet and Health*, and reports on disease prevention prepared by the National Academy of Sciences and the American Heart Association.

In general, macrobiotic dietary guidelines suggest:

Eating More	Eating Less
Complex carbohydrates	Simple sugars
Vegetable proteins	Animal proteins
Low-fat foods	High-fat foods
Low or no-cholesterol foods	High-cholesterol foods
Organically grown foods	Foods that have been chemically sprayed or fertilized
Naturally processed foods	Artificial or chemically processed foods
Whole foods	Refined and partial foods
Foods rich in fiber	Foods that have been devitalized

with these new foods. Breakfast, for example, is often more simple, consisting of a whole grain porridge, miso soup, and a few basic side dishes, while lunch and dinner can be more elaborate. However, we do suggest that whole grains form the main food at each meal and that you have adequate variety in your daily diet as a whole. The recipes found in the following chapters can help you get started with a wide range of foods and translate these guidelines into delicious and nourishing breakfasts.

Principal foods (the macrobiotic "four food groups") are generally eaten daily and include whole grains, beans and bean products, vegetables, and sea vegetables. Low-fat white-meat fish, seasonal fruits, natural desserts, nuts, seeds, natural sweeteners, and other supplementary foods are eaten less often, while condiments, pickles, snacks, seasonings, and beverages can be used daily, but in smaller quantities than principal foods. In order to help you in selecting the most appropriate foods for breakfast, we have added special recommendations at the end of each category.

STANDARD MACROBIOTIC DIET

The standard macrobiotic way of eating offers an incredible variety of foods and cooking methods from which to choose. The guidelines that follow are broad and flexible. You can apply them when selecting the highest-quality natural foods for your breakfasts and other meals. Refer to Figure 2.1, which details the standard macrobiotic diet.

Whole Cereal Grains

Whole cereal grains are the staff of life and an essential part of a balanced diet. If you live in a temperate climate, they may compose as much as 50 to 60 percent of your daily intake. Below is a list of the whole grains and grain products that may be included in your diet.

Sweet Brown Rice
Sweet brown rice grain
Mochi (pounded sweet rice)
Sweet brown rice flour products

Millet
Millet grain
Millet flour products
Puffed millet

Barley
Barley grain
Pearl barley
Puffed barley
Barley flour products

Rye
Rye grain
Rye bread
Rye flakes
Rye flour products

Buckwheat
Buckwheat groats (kasha)
Buckwheat noodles (soba) and
  pastas
Buckwheat flour products such as
  pancakes

Brown Rice
Brown rice—short, medium, and
  long grain
Genuine brown rice cream
Puffed brown rice
Brown rice flakes

Corn
Corn on the cob
Corn grits
Cornmeal
Arepas
Corn flour products such as bread
  and muffins
Puffed corn
Popped corn

Oats
Whole oats
Steel-cut oats
Rolled oats
Oatmeal
Oat flakes
Oat flour products

Whole Wheat
Whole wheat berries
Whole wheat bread
Whole wheat chapatis
Whole wheat noodles and
  pastas
Whole wheat flakes
Whole wheat flour
Whole wheat flour products
  such as crackers, matzos, and
  muffins
Couscous
Bulgur
Fu (baked puffed wheat gluten)
Seitan (wheat gluten)

Cooked whole grains are preferable to flour products or to cracked or rolled grains because of easier digestibility. In general, it is better to keep the intake of flour products—or cracked or rolled grains—less than 15 to 20 percent of your daily consumption of whole grains.

Special Considerations for Breakfast. Although leftover grains can be served as is for breakfast, soft porridges made from whole grains themselves, rather than from ground or crushed cereals, are preferred. Whole grain porridges can be made from scratch, by cooking grains with more water than usual, or by adding water to leftover grain dishes and cooking them for a short time, Flaked cereals, including rolled oats, barley flakes, and rye flakes, are less preferable than porridges made from whole grains. When eaten excessively, these foods can cause mucus to accumulate in the body; however, persons in good health can enjoy them from time to time for variety.

For optimal health, flour products such as pancakes, waffles, and muffins are best enjoyed only on special occasions. Breads, such as natural sourdough and whole wheat, can be eaten from time to time and are best when steamed. Steamed bread is soft and moist and is appropriate for harmonizing our condition with the light, rising energy of the morning. Toasted bread should be avoided due to its dry, contracting

Figure 2.1 The Standard Macrobiotic Diet

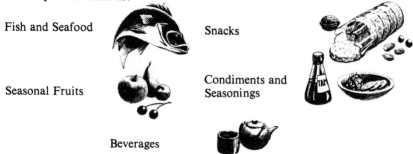

Whole Cereal
Grains 50–60%

Soup
5%

Vegetables
25–30%

Beans and
Sea Vegetables
5–10%

Plus Supplementary Foods such as:

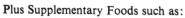

Fish and Seafood

Snacks

Seasonal Fruits

Condiments and
Seasonings

Beverages

nature. It can produce hardness and stagnation in the body. It should only be eaten occasionally and only by those in good overall health. Pounded sweet rice dumplings and mochi are also delicious at breakfast and can be added to morning miso soup.

Soups

Soups may compose about 5 percent of your daily intake. For most people, that averages out to about one or two cups per day. A wide variety of ingredients, including vegetables, grains, beans, sea vegetables, noodles, tofu, tempeh, and occasionally fish or seafood are wonderful in soups. Soups are delicious when moderately seasoned with either miso, tamari soy sauce, sea salt, umeboshi plum or paste, or ginger.

Soups can be made thick and rich, or as simple clear broths. Vegetable, grain, or bean stews can also be enjoyed, while a variety of garnishes, such as scallions, parsley, nori sea vegetable, and croutons, may be used to enhance their appearance and flavor.

One small bowl or cup of light miso soup with vegetables and wakame or kombu is recommended daily. Barley (mugi) miso is the best for regular consumption, followed by soybean (hatcho) miso. (More information on miso soup can be found beginning on page 83.) A second cup or bowl of soup may also be enjoyed, preferably mildly seasoned with tamari soy sauce or sea salt. Other healthful varieties of soup include:

> Bean and vegetable soups
> Grain and vegetable soups
> Puréed squash and other vegetable soups

Special Considerations for Breakfast.   Light miso or tamari soy sauce soups are ideal at breakfast. They complement the thick, creamy quality of whole grain porridges. Although rich soups and stews are quite nourishing and delicious, they may be a little too heavy in the morning, and are more enjoyable at lunch or dinner, when a greater variety of side dishes are included.

Soup flavored lightly with barley miso is especially good at breakfast. Miso is a dark purée made from soybeans, unrefined sea salt, and fermented barley or rice. It is traditionally prepared without chemicals by allowing the ingredients to ferment slowly in wooden kegs. The energy of natural fermentation matches the light, rising energy of morning. Moreover, among the cereal grains, barley is especially noted for its light and expansive qualities, making it an ideal breakfast food. Miso soup is also good for digestion and is perfect for activating the digestive system in the morning.

Vegetables

Roughly 25 to 30 percent of your daily intake can include vegetables. Nature provides an incredible variety of fresh local vegetables to choose from.

Recommended for Regular Use

Acorn squash
Bok choy
Broccoli
Burdock root
Buttercup squash
Butternut squash
Cabbage
Celery
Celery root
Carrots
Carrot tops
Cauliflower
Chinese cabbage
Chives
Collard greens
Cucumbers
Daikon
Daikon greens
Dandelion greens
Dandelion root
Endive
Escarole
Green beans
Green peas
Hubbard squash
Hokkaido pumpkin
Iceberg lettuce

Jinenjo (Japanese
   mountain potato)
Jerusalem artichokes
Kale
Kohlrabi
Leeks
Lotus root
Mushrooms
Mustard greens
Onions
Parsley
Parsnips
Pumpkin
Pattypan squash
Radishes
Red cabbage
Romaine lettuce
Scallions
Shiitake (dried Japan-
   ese) mushrooms
Snap beans
Summer squash
Turnips
Turnip greens
Watercress
Wax beans

Avoid for Optimal Health

Artichokes
Bamboo shoots
Beets
Curly dock
Eggplant
Fennel
Ferns
Ginseng

Green/red pepper
New Zealand spinach
Okra
Plantain
Potatoes
Purslane
Shepherd's purse
Sorrel

Spinach   Tomatoes
Sweet potatoes   Yams
Swiss chard   Zucchini
Taro (albi) potatoes

Vegetables can be served in soups or with grains, beans, or sea vegetables. They can also be used in making rice rolls (homemade sushi), served with noodles or pasta, cooked with fish, or served alone. The most common methods for cooking vegetables include boiling, steaming, pressing, sautéing (both waterless and with oil), and pickling. A variety of natural seasonings, including miso, tamari soy sauce, sea salt, and brown rice or umeboshi vinegar, are recommended in vegetable cookery. Vegetables from tropical climates are not recommended for use in the temperate zones, nor are nightshade vegetables such as tomatoes, potatoes, and eggplant. Three to five vegetable side dishes can be prepared daily to ensure adequate variety.

Special Considerations for Breakfast.   A wide variety of vegetables can be used in your breakfast dishes. Vegetable side dishes can be prepared according to your desires and preferences; however, cooking methods such as quick-steaming, boiling, sautéing, or pickling accentuate upward energy and are often most suitable in the morning. Green leafy vegetables are especially good when prepared using these methods. Vegetables are also delicious in soups and whole grain porridges. Daikon, squash, and cabbage add a wonderfully sweet taste to soft rice and other whole grain porridges. Raw scallions, parsley, and chives are strongly charged with upward energy and can be used often as garnishes for soups, porridges, and other dishes.

Beans

About 5 to 10 percent of your daily diet may include beans, peas, or bean products. Select from any of the varieties listed below:

Beans and Peas   Mung beans
Azuki beans   Navy beans
Bean sprouts   Pinto beans
Black-eyed peas   Soybeans
Black soybeans   Split peas
Chickpeas (garbanzo beans)   Whole dried peas
Great Northern beans
Kidney beans   **Bean Products**
Lentils (green and red)   Dried tofu (soybean curd that
Lima beans   has been naturally dried)

Fresh tofu
Natto (fermented soybeans)
Okara (pulp or residue left
from making tofu)

Tempeh (fermented soy-
beans or combination of
soybeans and grains)
Yuba (dried soymilk)

Beans and bean products are more easily digested when cooked with a small volume of seasonings such as sea salt, miso, or kombu sea vegetable. They may also be prepared with vegetables, chestnuts, dried apples, or raisins, and occasionally sweetened with grain sweeteners such as barley malt and rice honey. Serve them in soups and side dishes or with grains or sea vegetables.

Special Considerations for Breakfast. Beans are generally higher in fat and protein than grains and can be difficult to digest the first thing in the morning. They are not featured very often in macrobiotic breakfast menus, but are used more for lunch or dinner. Fermented soybean foods, such as tofu, dried tofu, and tempeh, are generally easier to digest and can be included more often at breakfast. (The natural fermentation used in making these foods can be thought of as a form of predigestion.) These fermented soy foods provide an excellent source of low-fat, no-cholesterol protein.

Sea Vegetables

Sea vegetables provide essential minerals and may be used daily in cooking. Arame and hijiki make wonderful side dishes and can be eaten several times per week. Wakame and kombu can be used daily in miso and other soups, in vegetable and bean dishes, or in making condiments. Toasted nori is a good source of iron and is also recommended for daily or regular use. Agar-agar can be used from time to time in making a natural jellied dessert known as kanten. See the inset beginning on page 86 for further information on sea vegetables.

Commonly Used Sea Vegetables

Arame	Kombu
Agar-agar	Mekabu
Dulse	Nekabu
Hijiki	Nori
Irish moss	Wakame

Special Considerations for Breakfast. Wakame and nori are generally lighter than the other sea vegetables and are used most often at breakfast. Wakame can be included in morning miso soup and lightly toasted nori can be used as a garnish for soups and porridges. Hijiki and arame are used to make side dishes that are usually served at dinner. Kombu can be used as a seasoning in whole grain porridges and as a base for soup broths and stocks. Wakame and kombu are also used in making condiments that can be sprinkled on porridge and other breakfast foods to add taste and nutrients.

Fish and Seafood

Fish and seafood can be eaten on occasion to supplement the foods previously discussed. Amounts eaten can vary, depending upon individual needs and desires. Generally, it is acceptable to eat fish and seafood several times per week as part of a balanced meal. White-meat varieties are lowest in saturated fat and are most easily digested; these are best for regular use.

Regular Use

Carp	Small dried fish
Cod	(iriko)
Flounder	Smelt
Haddock	Snapper
Halibut	Sole
Herring	Trout
Scrod	Other white-meat fish

Occasional Use

Infrequent Use

Cherrystone clams	Bluefish
Crabs	Salmon
Littleneck clams	Sardines
Lobster	Swordfish
Oysters	Tuna
Shrimp	Other blue-skinned and
	red-meat fish

Garnishes are especially important in balancing fish and seafood. Recommended garnishes include: chopped scallions or parsley, grated or shredded raw daikon, ginger, radish or horseradish, wasabi (green mustard paste), and raw salad.

Special Considerations for Breakfast. In general, fish and seafood contain too much protein and fat for regular use in the morning, although people in far-northern climates have traditionally enjoyed them for breakfast. Smoked salmon (lox) and other smoked or dried fish are very salty and contracting and can offset the smooth flow of upward energy in the body. Although fish and seafood are generally best eaten at other meals, they can be included, once in a while, for special-occasion breakfasts.

Fruit

In most cases, fruit can be enjoyed three or four times per week. Locally grown or temperate-climate fruits are preferable; tropical fruits are not recommended for regular use by people in temperate regions. Some of the varieties of fruit for consumption in temperate climates are listed below.

Recommended in a Temperate Climate

Apples	Peaches
Apricots	Persimmons
Blackberries	Plums
Cantaloupe	Raisins
Grapes	Raspberries
Honeydew	Strawberries
melon	Tangerines
Lemons	Watermelon
Mulberries	Wild berries

Avoid in a Temperate Climate

Bananas
Dates
Figs
Pineapple
Other tropical or
  semitropical fruits

Special Considerations for Breakfast.   Compared with whole grains, beans, and land and sea vegetables, fruits contain much smaller amounts of complex carbohydrates, fiber, protein, unsaturated fat, and essential vitamins and minerals. Most of their composition is water. Fructose, the primary carbohydrate in fruit, is a simple sugar and enters the bloodstream more rapidly than the complex sugars found in grains and vegetables. The energy fruits give is very light and expansive and needs to be balanced by the strong centering energy of these other types of food in order to maintain health and vitality. In general, fruits are not included in macrobiotic breakfasts on a regular basis. They are used on special occasions. Dried fruits such as raisins or apples can be added to porridge, while apple or other cooked purées are used as toppings for whole grain pancakes or waffles.

Many fruits, including the more extreme tropical varieties such as bananas, dates, and citrus, have become popular in modern breakfasts to provide balance for fatty, oily, and greasy foods. However, this balance is, on the whole, more extreme and can lead to a variety of health problems.

Pickles

Pickles can be eaten frequently as a supplement to main dishes. They stimulate appetite and help digestion. Some varieties—such as pickled daikon, or takuan—can be bought prepackaged in natural foods stores. Others, such as "quick pickles," can be prepared at home.

Regular Use	Avoid
Amazake pickles	Dill pickles
Brine pickles	Garlic pickles
Miso pickles	Herb pickles
Pressed pickles	Spiced pickles
Rice bran pickles	Vinegar pickles
Sauerkraut	
Takuan pickles	
Tamari soy sauce pickles	

Special Considerations for Breakfast.   Quick, light pickles are often eaten for breakfast in the Far East along with rice and miso soup. Their naturally fermented quality is generally in accord with the rising energy of morning and they help activate digestion. Pickles that are fermented for a shorter amount of time are generally preferred for use at breakfast, while those aged for longer times are better at other meals. A small serving of pickles can be included several times per week in macrobiotic breakfasts.

Seeds and Nuts

Seeds and nuts can be eaten from time to time as snacks and garnishes. They can be roasted with or without sea salt, sweetened with barley or rice malt, or seasoned with tamari soy sauce. Seeds and nuts can be ground into butter, shaved and served as garnishes or toppings, and can be used in a variety of dishes, including desserts. Different varieties of seeds and nuts are listed on the next page.

Nuts (Regular Use)
Almonds
Chestnuts
Filberts
Peanuts
Pecans
Pine nuts
Small Spanish nuts
Walnuts

Nuts (Occasional Use)
Brazil nuts
Cashews
Macadamia nuts

Seeds (Regular Use)
Pumpkin seeds
Sesame seeds (black and white)
Squash seeds

Seeds (Occasional Use)
Alfalfa seeds
Poppy seeds
Sunflower seeds
Umeboshi plum seeds

Special Considerations for Breakfast. Nuts are generally too high in fat and oil for use at breakfast. However, lightly roasted seeds are sometimes used as garnishes for porridge and other breakfast dishes. Naturally processed sesame seed butter can also be used, on occasion, as a natural spread on whole grain bread.

Snacks

A variety of natural snacks may be enjoyed from time to time, including those made from whole grains, such as cookies, bread, puffed cereals, mochi (pounded sweet brown rice), popcorn (homemade and unbuttered), rice cakes, rice balls, and homemade sushi. Lightly roasted nuts and seeds may also be eaten as snacks.

Special Considerations for Breakfast. As we mentioned in our discussion of grains, steamed whole grain bread is easily digestible and well suited for breakfast. Mochi, or pounded sweet brown rice, is also a wonderful breakfast food and can often be added to miso soup. Puffed whole grain cereals, including brown rice, whole wheat, barley, millet, and whole corn, can be enjoyed from time to time along with amazake, a naturally fermented sweet rice milk. Of course, many breakfast dishes incorporate leftovers from other meals. For example, quick porridges can be made from leftover grains; leftover soups can be simply reheated and enjoyed for breakfast.

Condiments

A variety of condiments may be used, some daily and others occasionally. Small amounts can be sprinkled on foods to adjust taste and nutritional value, and to stimulate appetite. They can be used on grains, soups, vegetables, beans, and sometimes desserts. The most frequently used varieties are listed below.

Condiments (Regular Use)

Gomashio (roasted sesame seeds and sea salt)

Green nori flakes

Sea-vegetable powders (with or without roasted sesame seeds)

Tekka (a special condiment made with soybean miso, sesame oil, burdock, lotus root, carrots, and ginger)

Umeboshi plums

Condiments (Occasional Use)

Roasted sesame seeds

Roasted and chopped shiso (pickled beefsteak plant) leaves

Shio kombu (kombu cooked with tamari and water)

Cooked nori condiment

Cooked miso with scallions or onions

Umeboshi or brown rice vinegar

Special Considerations for Breakfast.   Any of the regularly used condiments can be enjoyed on breakfast porridges. Fresh gomashio and sea-vegetable powders are especially delicious when sprinkled on brown rice, whole oat, or other hot breakfast cereals. Many people prefer to use stronger condiments, such as umeboshi plums, tekka, and nori condiment, at lunch or dinner when a wider variety of side dishes are served. Condiments such as mustard and ketchup are usually processed with refined sugar and are best avoided.

Seasonings

It is best to avoid strong, spicy seasonings such as curry and hot pepper. Instead, use only mild seasonings that have been naturally processed from vegetable products or natural sea salt. Many of these seasonings have been used as a part of traditional diets for many years. A list of such seasonings is presented below.

Seasonings for Regular Use

Unrefined sea salt

Soy sauce

Tamari soy sauce (fermented soybean and grain sauce)

Miso (fermented soybean and grain paste)

Brown rice and umeboshi vinegar

Barley malt and rice syrup

Grated daikon, radish, and ginger

Umeboshi plum and paste

Lemon, tangerine, and orange juice

Green and yellow mustard paste

Sesame, corn, safflower, mustard seed, and olive oil

Mirin (fermented sweet brown rice sweetener)

Amazake (fermented sweet brown rice beverage)

Seasonings to Avoid
Commercial seasonings
Stimulant and aromatic spices and herbs
Irradiated spices and herbs

Special Considerations for Breakfast.   As much as possible, seasonings are used to bring forth the naturally sweet taste of whole grains, beans, vegetables, and other complex carbohydrate foods. We therefore recommend using them moderately to season your breakfast porridges and other dishes. Pepper, spices, and other stimulating seasonings create overactive energy in the body and are used primarily as balance for extremely contractive animal foods. Generally, they should be avoided in macrobiotic breakfasts. Oil can be used, on occasion, when sautéing vegetables and other dishes; however, it is difficult to digest in the morning and should not be used regularly.

Garnishes

A variety of garnishes can be used to create balance among dishes and facilitate digestion. The use of garnishes depends upon the needs and desires of each person.

Commonly Used Garnishes
Grated daikon (for fish, mochi, and noodles)
Grated radish (use like grated daikon)
Grated horseradish (use mostly for fish or seafood)
Chopped scallions (for noodles, fish, and seafood)
Parsley
Lemon, tangerine, and orange slices (mainly for fish and seafood)

Special Considerations for Breakfast.   Garnishes add a light, upward energy to breakfast dishes and help harmonize them with the environment of morning. Chopped scallions or parsley are used frequently to garnish morning miso soups, porridges, and other breakfast dishes. In general, macrobiotic garnishes are kept simple and elegant.

Desserts and Sweets

A variety of natural desserts may be eaten from time to time, usually at the end of the main meal. Desserts can be made from azuki beans (sweetened with grain syrup, chestnuts, squash, or raisins); cooked or dried fruit; agar-agar (natural sea-vegetable gelatin); grains (e.g., rice pudding, couscous cake, and Indian pudding); and flour products (cookies, cakes, pies, and muffins) prepared with fruit or grain sweeteners.

The naturally sweet flavor of cooked vegetables can be featured daily for optimal health. Include one or several of the vegetables listed below.

For Regular Use

Cabbage	Parsnips
Carrots	Pumpkin
Daikon	Squash
Onions	

In addition, a small amount of concentrated sweeteners made from whole cereal grains may be included when desired. Dried chestnuts, which impart a sweet flavor, may also be included on occasion, as well as apple juice or cider. Additional natural sweeteners are listed below.

Common Natural Sweeteners

Amazake	Hot apple cider
Barley malt	Hot apple juice
Brown rice syrup	Mirin
Chestnuts (cooked)	

Special Considerations for Breakfast. Naturally sweet vegetables are used often in macrobiotic breakfast dishes. Onion, squash, cabbage, and carrots add a wonderful sweetness to morning miso soup. They can also be cooked in with whole grain porridges for additional sweetness. Squash purée can be used as a topping for porridges, steamed bread, or special occasion waffles and pancakes. Amazake, or sweet rice milk, can sometimes be used in porridge for an added touch of sweetness, as can a small amount of rice syrup or barley malt. Naturally processed grain sweeteners are preferred over maple syrup or honey as a topping for whole grain pancakes and waffles.

Beverages

A variety of beverages may be consumed daily or occasionally. Amounts can vary according to each person's needs and the weather conditions. The following beverages can be used to comfortably satisfy the desire for liquid.

Beverages for Regular Use

Bancha twig and stem tea
Roasted brown rice or barley tea
Cereal grain coffee
Spring or well water
Amazake
Dandelion tea
Soybean milk (prepared with kombu)
Kombu tea
Lotus root tea
Mu tea
Sake (fermented rice wine, without chemicals or sugar)
Beer (brewed naturally, without sugar or additives)
Apple, grape, or apricot juices
Apple cider
Carrot, celery, and other vegetable juices

Beverages to Avoid

Distilled water
Coffee
Cold or iced drinks
Hard liquor
Aromatic herbal teas
Mineral water and all bubbling waters
Chemically colored tea
Stimulant beverages
Sugared drinks
Tap water
Tropical fruit juices
Chemically processed beverages

Special Considerations for Breakfast. For many people caffeine-free, bancha twig tea is the beverage of choice at breakfast, followed by barley, brown rice, and other whole grain teas. Cereal grain coffees can also be enjoyed, on occasion, by those in good overall health. Soymilk is too high in fat for regular use, and is best reserved for special occasions.

NATURAL LIFESTYLE SUGGESTIONS

Macrobiotics is far more than just a diet. It encompasses a whole lifestyle aimed at re-establishing our connection with nature. Together with eating well, a number of practices are recommended for health and well-being. Practices such as keeping physically active and using natural cooking utensils, fabrics, and materials in the home are especially recommended. In the past, people lived more closely with nature and ate a more balanced, natural diet. With each generation, we have gotten further and further from our roots in nature, and have experienced a corresponding decline in health. The suggestions presented below complement a balanced, natural diet and can help you enjoy more satisfying and harmonious living.

- Live each day happily without being worried about your health. Keep active mentally and physically. Sing every day and encourage others to join with you.
- Greet everyone and everything with gratitude. In particular, offer thanks before and after each meal. Encourage others to give thanks for their food and their natural environment.
- Try to get to bed before midnight and get up early in the morning.
- Try not to wear synthetic clothing or woolen articles directly against your skin. Wear cotton instead. Keep jewelry and accessories simple, natural, and graceful.
- If you are able, go outdoors in simple clothing every day. When the weather permits, walk barefoot on the grass, the soil, or the beach. Go on regular outings, especially to beautiful, natural areas.
- Keep your home shiny clean and orderly. Keep the atmosphere of your home bright and cheerful.
- Maintain an active correspondence. Express love and appreciation to your parents, husband or wife, children, brothers, sisters, relatives, friends, and associates.
- Try not to take long, hot baths or showers unless you have been consuming too much salt or animal food.
- Every morning or every night, scrub your whole body with a hot, moist towel until your circulation becomes active. When a complete body scrub is not convenient, at least do your hands, feet, fingers, and toes.
- Use natural cosmetics, soaps, shampoos, and body care products. Brush your teeth with sea salt or other natural preparations, such as *denti* (roasted eggplant and sea salt).
- Keep as active as you can. Daily activities such as cooking, scrubbing floors, cleaning windows, and washing clothes are excellent forms of exercise. You may also try systematic exercise programs such as yoga, martial arts, aerobics, and sports. A daily half-hour walk is an especially good way to activate your energy and circulation.
- Try to minimize time spent in front of the television. Color TV, especially, emits unnatural radiation that can be physically draining. Turn the TV off during mealtimes. Balance television with more productive activities.
- Switch from electric to gas cooking at the earliest opportunity. Microwave cooking is best avoided.

- Heating pads, electric blankets, portable radios with earphones, and other electrical devices can disrupt the body's natural flow of energy. They are not recommended for regular use.
- Put many green plants throughout your house to freshen and enrich the air.

The way we eat can be just as important as our choice of foods. Regularly scheduled meals are best. Be sure to include a whole grain dish at each meal (the word "meal" actually means "crushed whole grain"). The amount of food eaten depends on your needs. Snacking should be kept to a minimum so that it doesn't replace meals, while tea and other beverages can be enjoyed throughout the day as desired. Chewing is also important; try to chew each mouthful of food until it becomes liquid. You can eat whenever you feel hungry, but try to avoid eating at least three hours before bedtime. Food eaten before sleeping often does not digest properly and can lead to indigestion and stagnation in the body.

As hundreds of thousands of people around the world have discovered, these basic guidelines can help restore and maintain optimal health. However, no matter how wonderful these dietary and lifestyle guidelines sound, the key is to apply them successfully. In the chapters that follow, we will show you how to translate these suggestions into appetizing and nourishing dishes that can help you begin your day healthfully and enjoyably.

Chapter Three
PRELIMINARIES

Macrobiotic breakfasts can be divided into three categories. The first is the *from-scratch breakfast*. In this meal, our main dishes are prepared fresh every morning. The whole grains used in porridge are washed and cooked in the morning; the vegetables for soup are washed, cut, and added to the broth; and each side dish is started from the beginning. Of course, things like condiments, pickles, and beverages are usually made beforehand, and can be incorporated into the meal.

The second type of breakfast is the *combination breakfast*. This usually features a mix of freshly made dishes and reheated leftovers from the previous day. Whole grains from the previous dinner are commonly used in making quick breakfast porridges. Simply add more water to them and reheat for a short time. A delicious, hot morning cereal will be the result. Miso and other soups can also be reheated from the previous day, although freshly made soups are especially delicious in the morning. Leftover vegetables can also be added to soup or porridge; they can also be reheated and eaten as is. Other leftovers can also be incorporated into breakfast.

The third type of breakfast is the *special-occasion breakfast*. This is traditionally reserved for Sunday mornings, when more time is available to prepare and enjoy special foods. This breakfast may include dishes that are not normally eaten during the week such as whole wheat waffles and pancakes, tofu "French toast," and scrambled tofu. How often you prepare special occasion breakfasts and the foods you include in them can be determined by your individual dietary needs and preferences.

When planning menus, remember that a light and simple breakfast is best for harmonizing your condition with the environment of the morning. Too many dishes can produce a full, stuck feeling. Also, remember that whole grains are the primary foods at all macrobiotic meals, including breakfast. A whole grain porridge or other whole grain dish can make up at least 50 percent of your meal. As shown in the previous chapter, miso or other light soups go well with whole grains at breakfast. When preparing breakfast soups, keep them light and simple. This means not using too many ingredients and keeping the use of miso or other seasonings mild.

The vegetable or other side dishes included should be selected according to individual health conditions, preferences, and the amount of time that is available. As stated, however, quickly steamed or boiled greens have a nice light energy that goes well with the rising energy of morning. Bean and sea vegetable side dishes are often too heavy in the morning and are usually served at other meals. Condiments such as gomashio and sea-vegetable powders can be used on porridges and other dishes, while bancha tea and cereal grain teas are often the most popular beverages at breakfast. On occasion, a small amount of amazake, concentrated grain sweetener, or raisins can be added to porridge for a naturally sweet flavor.

In the chapters that follow we present a wide variety of dishes that can be included in a healthful breakfast. We start with whole grains and porridges, and then describe a variety of morning miso and other soups. Also included are recipes for breakfast vegetables, as well as a description of how to make quick light pickles. In addition, recipes for preparing tempeh, tofu, and other soybean foods at breakfast are included, as well as suggestions for making and using condiments and beverages. We conclude the book with a chapter on special occasion breakfasts. Before we get started with the recipes, however, let us first consider some of the preliminary steps involved in cooking macrobiotically, beginning with the selection of the highest-quality cooking utensils and foods.

THE TOOLS OF THE TRADE

High-quality cookware can make the difference between a delicious breakfast and an average one, and can enhance or detract from the natural quality of the foods you cook. Below are some of the most essential items used in preparing breakfasts and other macrobiotic meals.

Pressure Cooker.   A stainless steel pressure cooker is an important utensil for preparing brown rice and other whole grains. A five-liter cooker is usually sufficient for recipes serving up to six people. There are many fine models to choose from. Ask the salesperson in your natural foods store for suggestions on the right model for your needs.

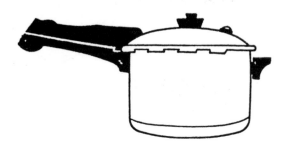

Pressure Cooker

Cookware. Stainless steel cookware is recommended for everyday use. Skillets made from cast iron are also fine for occasional use in sautéing and deep frying. Aluminum, teflon, and other non-stick coated cookware is not recommended if you wish to achieve optimum health. Aluminum is absorbed into food, while non-stick or plastic coatings are easily chipped, allowing minute particles from the surface to get into the food.

Cooking Utensils. Wooden utensils are fairly inexpensive and are made from a material that is harmonious with our everyday needs. Start with basic items such as soup ladles, bamboo rice paddles, a roasting paddle, spoons of various sizes, and cooking chopsticks. Metal tableware is fine if you prefer it, although many people like to use chopsticks and ceramic or wooden spoons, since they prefer the natural feel of wood or clay.

Knives. A high-grade stainless or carbon steel knife is recommended for efficient cutting. Keep your knife properly sharpened, as this can make the difference between smooth, quick cutting and spending unnecessary time in the kitchen. Electric knives and food processors are generally not recommended, as the use of electricity disrupts the natural balance and energy of food.

Cutting Board. A high-quality wooden cutting board is helpful for cutting vegetables and other foods. You may want to purchase two: a larger one for vegetable foods, and a smaller one for fish and seafood.

Flame Deflector. Flame deflectors are metal pads that are placed under pressure cookers and other pots to distribute heat evenly and prevent burning. Metal deflectors are available at natural foods stores as well as variety stores.

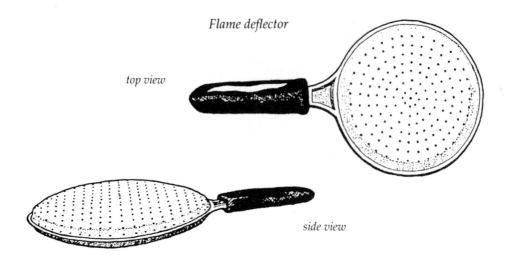

Flame deflector

top view

side view

Natural Bristle Brushes.   Small brushes with natural bristles are recommended for cleaning vegetables. They are especially good for scrubbing roots like carrots and burdock, and are available in natural foods stores and kitchen specialty shops.

Containers.   Glass, ceramic, or wooden containers are recommended for storing dried foods. Unlike plastic or metal, they do not change the smell or taste of foods. These containers and jars come in many shapes and sizes and can be purchased as needed.

Tamari Dispensers.   These specially made small glass bottles are used to store tamari soy sauce for handy use. The dispensers make it easy to control the flow of tamari when you add it to food during cooking.

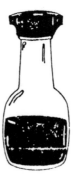

Tamari soy sauce dispenser

Strainers and Colanders.   A wire mesh strainer or colander is useful for washing and rinsing foods. Large mesh strainers are appropriate for most items, while fine mesh varieties are better for smaller grains and seeds. A bamboo tea strainer is also very useful when straining tea into cups. These items are available at many natural foods stores.

Graters. Of the several types of graters available, the most useful is a flat metal vegetable grater. It is convenient for grating daikon, ginger root, and other vegetables. Other types of graters can also be useful in preparing dishes like sauerkraut, or in making salads.

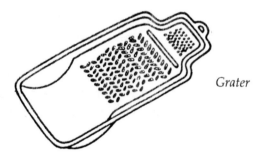

Grater

Suribachi. These small Japanese grinding bowls are made of clay and are useful in making gomashio and other condiments, as well as in making sauces, dips, and salad dressings. They are also helpful when purée-ing foods. They come with a small wood pestle known as a surikogi, and are available in natural foods stores.

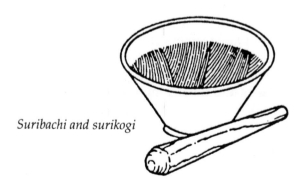

Suribachi and surikogi

Pickle Press. This plastic utensil is very useful when preparing quick pickles and pressed salads. Pickle presses are available in many natural foods stores. If you can't locate one you can make pressed salads by placing the cut vegetables in a bowl, putting a plate or saucer on top, and adding a rock or weight of some sort to apply pressure. More detailed information on pickle presses can be found under the *Pressing* section in Chapter Six.

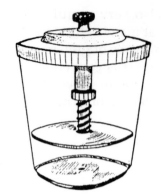

Pickle press

Bamboo Sushi Mats. These flexible mats are made from thin strips of bamboo that are connected with string. They are handy to use when making macrobiotic sushi or for covering dishes of leftovers. It is a good idea to purchase several.

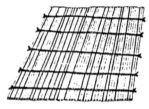

Bamboo sushi mat

Steamers. The most popular steamers are the collapsible stainless steel variety that fits inside cooking pots, and the bamboo type consisting of several layers that are stacked on a steaming pot of water. Steamers are handy for warming leftovers and for steaming greens and other foods.

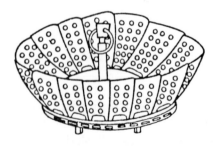

Stainless steel steamer

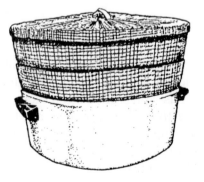

Bamboo steamer

Sharpening Stone. Keeping your vegetable knives properly sharpened makes cooking more enjoyable. The stones for sharpening knives are available at most hardware stores, natural foods stores, and kitchen specialty shops. When purchasing knives, ask the salesperson for sharpening instructions.

A BASIC SHOPPING LIST

When buying natural foods, it is important to select from among the highest-quality natural and organic products. Selecting a store that maintains high standards of quality is, therefore, essential. This is especially important when shopping for items such as grains, beans, sea vegetables, miso, tamari, sea salt, oils, umeboshi plums, seeds, noodles, and breads.

It is best to purchase organic vegetables, but in some cases it may not be possible. If you have difficulty locating organic produce and you have the space, you should think about starting your own vegetable garden. Organic seeds are available by mail from several seed companies in North America. When necessary, your organic staples can be supplemented with nonorganic produce from local markets. Nonorganic produce should be thoroughly washed and properly cooked to reduce potentially toxic residues.

You may choose to stock your pantry with new foods gradually or all at once. Embarking on a new way of cooking and eating can be fun and exciting. There are natural and macrobiotic foods stores in most cities and towns in the United States where you can shop. Several larger distributors have mail-order catalogues if you have trouble finding certain items.

Foods can be purchased in small quantities to suit individual or family needs or in larger bulk quantities at reduced prices. Below is a basic list of staple items that are used in making breakfasts and other meals. As you purchase them, these items can be stored in glass, ceramic, or wooden containers, and, in some cases, in the refrigerator.

Grains. Brown rice (short grain is suitable for four-season climates, while for warmer climates you may also want to use medium grain), barley, pearl barley, (sometimes sold under the name *hato mugi*), millet, sweet brown rice, rolled oats, whole oats, wheat berries, kasha (buckwheat), fresh corn in season, and whole rye. Cracked or partially refined grains may be purchased for occasional use. These include bulgur, cracked wheat, and couscous.

Noodles. Whole wheat noodles, (including udon and somen); soba (buckwheat noodles); whole wheat pasta and spaghetti; whole wheat rice, and buckwheat ramen.

Beans. Azuki beans, lentils, chickpeas, black soybeans, white soybeans, black turtle beans, kidney beans, pinto beans, navy beans, Great Northern beans, split peas, whole green peas, and lima beans.

Sea Vegetables.   Arame, hijiki, nori, kombu, wakame, dulse, sea palm, agar-agar, and kelp.

Condiments and Seasonings.   Barley miso, hatcho miso, tamari soy sauce, umeboshi plums, umeboshi paste, umeboshi vinegar, brown rice vinegar, ginger root, barley malt, rice syrup, sweet brown rice vinegar, hato mugi vinegar, mirin (a sweet rice cooking wine), and sea salt.

Other condiments can be prepared at home and kept in tightly sealed glass containers. Homemade condiments are fresher than store-bought varieties, and the ingredients can be specially balanced to suit your personal needs. Homemade varieties include gomashio (black or tan), goma wakame, kombu powder, shiso, shio nori, and shio kombu.

Beverages.   Bancha tea, roasted barley tea, and cereal grain coffee.

Seeds and Nuts.   Sesame (black and tan), sunflower, and pumpkin seeds. Dried chestnuts, walnuts, almonds, and roasted peanuts.

Flour and Flour Products.   Whole wheat bread and pastry flour, buckwheat and corn flour, and cornmeal. Whole wheat, sourdough, and rice bread can be eaten occasionally.

Dried Fruits.   Raisins, apples, apricots, currants, cherries, peaches, and pears.

Oils.   Unrefined dark sesame oil, light sesame oil, and corn oil.

Others.   Special items you might wish to stock include kuzu, arrowroot flour, dried tofu, amazake, shiitake mushrooms (dried Japanese mushrooms), snacks (rice cakes, puffed cereals, popping corn), dried daikon, fu, fresh tofu, tempeh, and dried lotus seeds (both white and red).

Perishable items such as fresh vegetables, fresh fruits, and tofu can be purchased as needed and stored in the refrigerator when necessary.

A KITCHEN PRIMER

With your cupboards and refrigerator stocked with high-quality natural foods, you are now ready to try your hand at cooking healthful breakfasts. Before you actually begin, it is important to be well prepared. Proper preparation saves time and energy, and gives you more freedom to be creative and apply your natural intuition and sense of balance. We would like to recommend the following practices as you begin cooking:

- Select your materials wisely from organic products naturally grown, in season, and from the climate or region in which you live.
- Try to use whole natural foods that are fresh until the time they are cooked.
- When cutting vegetables or other foods, prepare them individually and place each separately; avoid mixing vegetables until you begin to cook them. Also, wipe your cutting board clean after cutting each vegetable.

- Try to cut your vegetables as elegantly and gracefully as possible so
d.
w the flavors of the foods to mix together
them unnecessarily.
ely. Unrefined sea salt, cold-pressed veg-
sweeteners, whole grain vinegar and other
can be used to enhance the natural flavor
soning is kept mild.
ater for cooking and drinking—clean well,
water. City water can be used for washing
oid distilled water.
re usually not recommended in temperate

pealing by presenting them beautifully and
ors of foods can be harmonized through
nd attractive dishes.
ing area clean and orderly. Keep the atmos-
uiet and calm, and maintain a peaceful, lov-
d while cooking and eating.

COOKING FOOD

Proper cooking brings out and enhances the flavor of food, stimulates the appetite, and balances our condition with nature and the environment. By varying the selection of foods, cooking methods, cooking times, the water content of the various dishes, the cutting methods, and the seasonings used, the cook can continually build health and vitality, while adapting to the changing environment.

The cook's attitude also affects the quality of the meal being prepared. A calm peaceful mind is important while preparing and serving food. All distractions, problems, and stresses are best put aside when you enter the kitchen.

To cook in a natural, balanced way, it is important to be sensitive to the surrounding environment. Being aware of the changing seasons and learning how to adapt to them is necessary. For example, during the spring and summer it is better to use shorter cooking times and to serve light, fresh dishes. These help balance our condition with hotter weather. As we approach autumn and winter, our cooking should change to include more warming factors, such as a little more salt, oil, and other seasonings, and a greater number of hearty, well-cooked dishes like thick soups and stews. Daily weather conditions are also important. For example, on wet, rainy days, less water is needed in cooking; more can be added on dry, hot days.

The quality of fire used in cooking also plays a vital role in health and well-being. For most people, gas ranges are the most practical and healthful fuel source. They provide a clean, even, easily controllable flame. Many people who have changed to a natural diet have also converted from electric to gas cooking. Most report improvements in their cooking and the taste of their foods, as well as in their energy levels and overall health.

For those with electric stoves who are unable to install a gas range right away, small portable propane gas stoves can be used in the kitchen along with an electric range. These portable units have several burners, and can be used in preparing pressure-cooked rice, miso soup, and other staples, while side dishes can be prepared on the electric range.

Microwave ovens are not recommended for healthful cooking. Microwave cooking bombards food with radiation, the long-term effects of which are largely unknown. It cooks food rapidly from the inside out, rather than outside in, as a natural flame does. This rapidly expanding and explosive quality is similar to the rapid and uncontrollable growth of cells known as cancer.

WASHING FOODS

It is better not to wash and cut foods too soon before you are ready to use them, as this causes them to lose freshness and nutritional value. Wash vegetables before cutting them, because vegetables that are cut before being washed lose taste and nutrients.

Foods such as whole grains, beans, seeds, vegetables, sea vegetables, and fruits can be quickly washed with cold water. This causes the skin or shell of the food to contract and helps prevent nutrient loss. Foods washed with warm water are often bland tasting. Following are specific guidelines for washing various types of food.

Washing Grains, Beans, and Seeds.   Before washing these foods, first sort them to remove any small stones, clumps of soil, or badly damaged pieces. Place the grains, beans, or seeds in a bowl, put the bowl in the sink, and fill it with water beyond the level of the food. Stir gently with your fingers, then pour the water off. Repeat the process again, and then transfer the moist food, a handful at a time, to a strainer. Rinse quickly under cold water. Your grains, beans, or seeds are now ready to be cooked or roasted.

Washing Vegetables and Fruits.   Leafy green vegetables, especially those with jagged edges like kale and carrot greens, can be held under cold running water or soaked in a bowl of cold water for several seconds. An entire bunch of greens can be rinsed or soaked in this way. Then, wash each leaf by hand under cold running water. Most leafy greens require thorough washing before they are ready to be cooked. Larger leaves, like cabbage or Chinese cabbage, can be washed individually after they are separated from the core.

Root and round vegetables can be cleaned with a natural bristle vegetable brush, as can fruits. Scrub firmly but gently to remove soil. Be careful not to remove the skin while scrubbing. The skin of vegetables and fruits is best kept on, as it contains nutrients that are a part of the whole food. Onions are an exception; they can be peeled and quickly rinsed under cold water before slicing. Of course, produce that has been waxed or overly chemicalized requires peeling or at least thorough scrubbing.

Washing Sea Vegetables. Plants from the sea sometimes have tiny stones or shells attached to them; these are easy to remove by hand. Most sea vegetables can be washed in the manner described for grains and seeds. After washing, they should be soaked for about five minutes (until they become soft enough to slice smoothly). An exception to this is arame. This sea vegetable is shredded before being dried; it loses sweetness and flavor when it is soaked. It is better to simply wash arame and allow it to absorb the water that remains from washing. Also, kombu is normally wiped with a clean damp towel or sponge before soaking. Three to five minutes is normally all that is required when soaking most sea vegetables.

VEGETABLE CUTTING TECHNIQUES

A variety of cutting methods is recommended when cooking in order to create attractive and delicious dishes. As you familiarize yourself with the recipes in this book, you will discover that some dishes require thicker, more chunky-style cuts, while others require fine and delicate cuts. With practice, anyone can learn to cut vegetables in an artistic and balanced fashion.

When cutting vegetables, do not cut straight down or use your knife like a saw. Start with the front tip or edge, and gently slide the length of the blade across the vegetable in one smooth stroke. Keep your fingertips curled so that your knuckles rest against the knife. This protects against accidental cuts and slips and helps you get a better grip on the vegetable.

The basic cutting methods used in this book are illustrated in Figure 3.2. Additional cutting methods for vegetables and sea vegetables can be found on page 88.

CUTTING CORNERS

Once you begin cooking, you will discover many shortcuts to help save time and energy in the kitchen. One way to save time is to plan ahead so that all of the dishes in a meal are finished at the same time. Start the dishes that require the longest cooking time first, and those with shorter cooking times later. If, for example, your breakfast includes soft brown rice porridge, miso soup, steamed greens, and a quick-pressed salad, start the pressed salad first, as it needs to sit for an hour or so before it is ready. Then start your porridge, and move on to the miso

soup. Steamed greens take only a few minutes to cook and can be started last.

Once your dishes are cooking, you can save energy by letting the foods
cook themselves. Don't look into the cooking pots too often or stir your
foods unnecessarily. Simply check them now and then to make sure they
are cooking properly.

Figure 3.2   Cutting Methods

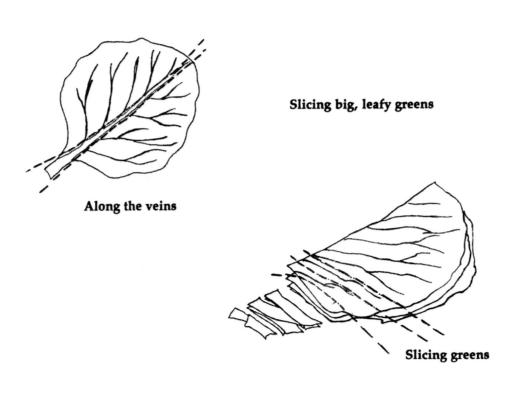

Slicing big, leafy greens

Along the veins

Slicing greens

The stem

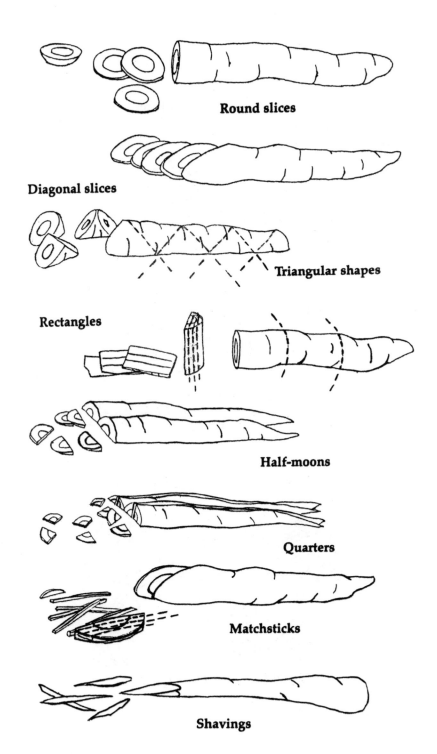

Round slices

Diagonal slices

Triangular shapes

Rectangles

Half-moons

Quarters

Matchsticks

Shavings

Cubes, dicing, and mincing

Wedge slices

Slicing cabbages

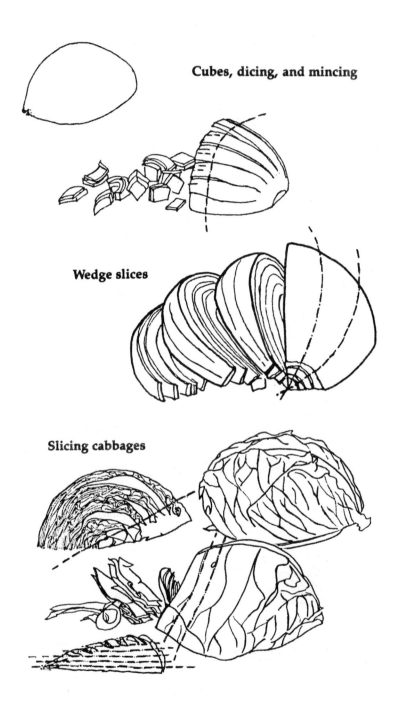

Chapter Four

WHOLE GRAINS AND PORRIDGES

Whole cereal grains have constituted the principal food of humanity for thousands of years. Every civilization prior to our own recognized whole grains as the staff of life. Whole cereal grains contain a balance of protein, carbohydrates, fat, and vitamins ideally suited for the human condition. Using them as principal foods helps secure a natural balance of energy and nutrients, and contributes to the maintenance of optimal health.

Complex carbohydrates found in whole grains are gradually and smoothly assimilated, providing a slow and steady source of energy to the body. Whole grains are also high in niacin and other B vitamins, vitamin E, and vitamin A. They are ideally suited as primary foods at breakfast and other meals. Soft breakfast porridges are the most commonly eaten breakfast cereals in macrobiotic households. In this chapter, we will explain how to make a variety of these soft and delicious breakfast cereals, and how to use whole grains in other ways at breakfast. Please refer to page 44 for instructions on washing whole grains prior to cooking.

BREAKFAST PORRIDGE PRELIMINARIES

How to Soak Whole Grains

Several of the grains with harder textures, such as whole wheat berries, rye, hulled barley, whole oats, and whole corn, become more digestible and require less cooking time if they are soaked prior to cooking. Softer grains, such as brown rice, hato mugi, millet, and sweet brown rice, usually don't need to be soaked.

To soak, place the washed grains in a bowl and cover with the amount of cold water specified in the recipe. Soak 6–8 hours or overnight. After soaking, place the grains and the soaking water in a pot or pressure cooker and follow the cooking instructions in the recipe.

How to Dry-Roast Whole Grains

From time to time, grain may be roasted prior to cooking in order to make it more contracted and energized. Roasting also reduces the amount of time needed to cook it, and produces grain dishes with light, dry, fluffy textures.

After washing and rinsing the grain, let it sit in a strainer for 2–3 minutes to drain, then place it in a heated skillet. Keep the flame at medium or medium-high at first, until much of the water from washing the grain evaporates. Take a wooden rice paddle or a wooden spoon, and gently, but constantly, move the grain back and forth in the skillet. Occasionally shake the skillet back and forth to move the grain from the bottom of the skillet to the top. This will help the grain to evenly roast and prevent it from burning. Reduce the flame to medium-low once the grain is dry and continue roasting until it is golden-brown. Be careful not to burn or scorch the grain, as this will cause it to have a bitter flavor when cooked. When the grain is finished, immediately remove it from the skillet. It is now ready to be cooked. Roasted grain can also be used to make delicious breakfast teas.

Using Leftover Grains

Leftover cooked grains can be reheated to make soft breakfast porridges or grain soups. It isn't necessary to add more salt if the grains were already cooked with it. If the grains were previously cooked with kombu, you can add a pinch of sea salt or a small amount of puréed miso for seasoning. To prepare soft porridge, simply place the leftover grain in a pot or a pressure cooker. Cover with cold water, place the lid on the pot, and boil for 20–25 minutes or pressure cook for 15–20 minutes.

Using Leftover Vegetables

Leftover vegetables, if kept in a cool place or are refrigerated to prevent spoilage, may be used, occasionally, in preparing breakfast porridge. If using leftover vegetables, you can add them at the very end of cooking, just long enough to heat them up, but not long enough to over-cook them. Over-cooking will produce bland-tasting, dull-colored, less-nutritious porridges.

Seasoning Breakfast Porridge

A variety of natural seasonings can be used when preparing breakfast porridge. Below is a list of recommended seasonings and guidelines for using them.

Miso. There are many types of miso to choose from, but the best for daily use to promote good health is barley miso (mugi miso). When using miso to season breakfast porridge, it must first be puréed in a small amount of liquid, and then added to the porridge after it has finished cooking. It is then simmered for 2–3 minutes on a low flame, so that the miso may evenly cook into the grain.

Sea Salt. Salt is added at the beginning when cooking grain, as it requires a longer cooking time to dissolve and thoroughly penetrate the grain. Uncooked or improperly cooked sea salt may produce a saltier-flavored dish and cause a more tightening effect in the body when eaten.

Kombu. Kombu sea vegetable is a mild, high-mineral, low-sodium seasoning that can be used by small children, for those on low-sodium diets, or for those who prefer a lighter, milder porridge. A small 1–1 1/2 inch piece of kombu is enough for each cup of uncooked grain. First, gently wipe off any dust with a clean, damp sponge. Then cover the kombu in cold water and soak for 3–5 minutes. Remove, slice or dice, and then add it to the washed grain at the beginning of cooking. The water that the kombu is soaked in is very mild and may be used as part of your water measurement.

Umeboshi Plums. These pickled, salty-sour plums are delicious when cooked in soft brown rice porridge. They can also be cooked with other grains as well. For 1 cup of uncooked grain, 1/2–1 small umeboshi plum is sufficient. The whole plum may be placed in the pot with the grain, at the beginning of cooking, or pulled apart and added in small pieces.

Tamari Soy Sauce. Tamari soy sauce is generally not used to prepare breakfast porridge, but may be used to mildly season fried grains and noodles, soups and broths, or lightly sautéed vegetables.

Dried Fruit. On special occasions, a small amount of dried apples, apricots, raisins, or other dried temperate-climate fruits may be used to sweeten breakfast porridge. However, dates, figs, dried bananas, pineapples, or other tropical or semitropical fruits are not recommended for optimal health. Dried fruits are usually added at the beginning and cooked along with the whole grains.

Whole Grain Sweeteners. Concentrated grain sweeteners such as brown rice syrup or barley malt can be used now and then for additional sweetness. They are easier to digest when cooked with porridge for several minutes, and are usually added near the end of cooking. Amazake (rice milk) is also delicious when poured over porridge and can be used on occasion.

Garnishes and Condiments

Garnishes help balance the energy in whole grains and other dishes. Macrobiotic condiments also add flavor and nutrients, and increase digestibility. Brightly colored garnishes complement the soft neutral color of grain dishes. Their varied flavors also create a balance for the naturally sweet flavor of whole grains. Choosing the right garnish to balance the flavor, texture, and color of your grain dishes is an important aspect of macrobiotic cooking. A list of macrobiotic condiments and garnishes for use at breakfast is presented in Table 4.1.

Cooking Methods for Soft-Grain Porridge

Basically, there are two methods of cooking soft-grain porridges: boiling and pressure cooking. But occasionally, for a richer, drier grain dish, you can pan-fry grains and noodles for breakfast.

Table 4.1   Breakfast Condiments and Garnishes

Condiment or Garnish	Flavor
Scallions (raw)	Pungent
Scallions (cooked)	Sweet
Chives	Pungent
Parsley	Bitter
Celery	Sour and bitter
Shiso	Sour and salty
Umeboshi	Sour and salty
Gomashio	Bitter and salty
Sea-vegetable powders	Bitter and salty
Nori flakes	Bitter and mildly salty
Toasted nori strips	Bitter and mildly salty
Miso condiments	Salty and sour
Roasted nuts	Bitter
Roasted nuts with salt	Bitter and salty
Roasted seeds	Bitter
Roasted seeds with salt	Bitter and salty
Raisins	Sweet
Dried fruit	Sweet (sometimes bitter or sour)
Grain sweeteners	Sweet
Amazake	Sweet and mildly sour

Boiling

Boiling is the most frequently used method of cooking whole grains for breakfast. Boiling is a slower, gentler, and less contracting method than pressure cooking or frying.

To prepare boiled grain porridge, place the washed grain in a heavy pot. Add water (usually 4–5 times the amount of grain; e.g., 1 cup of brown rice to 4–5 cups of water), and either a pinch of sea salt, a 1–1 1/2-inch strip of kombu, or a small umeboshi plum. (You may also choose to omit the seasoning entirely and add a condiment or garnish when served instead.) Then place the grains on a high flame, cover, and bring to a boil. Reduce the flame to medium-low and simmer for the amount of time indicated in the recipe. Place the soft porridge in serving bowls, garnish, and serve.

Pressure Cooking

Pressure cooking is the most commonly used method of preparing brown rice in most macrobiotic households. It makes brown rice sweeter and easier to digest, and prevents any nutrients from escaping in the steam. A common breakfast porridge is made by boiling leftover pressure-cooked brown rice from the night before. However, pressure cooking can also be used to prepare soft brown rice and other porridges from scratch in the morning. Pressure-cooked porridges are especially good in cold weather and when a heartier breakfast cereal is called for.

Place the washed grain in the pressure cooker, add the appropriate amount of water and seasoning, place the lid on the cooker, and put on a high flame. Bring up to pressure, reduce the flame to low, and simmer for the amount of time indicated in the recipe. Place cooked grains in individual serving bowls, garnish, and serve hot.

Pan-Frying

Fried foods are not used very often in macrobiotic breakfasts, as oil can be difficult to digest early in the morning. Fried grains are used more often in colder climates or seasons. Occasionally, this method is used in warmer weather if oil is needed to balance the strong, dry, summer sun, or if it is required for a dry, rich grain preparation. There are basically two ways to pan-fry grains or noodles:

With Water.   This method produces a moister dish. Brush a skillet with a small amount of light or dark sesame oil and heat up. Add sliced vegetables and sauté for 1–2 minutes. Place the leftover grain on top of the vegetables. Do not mix. Add several drops of cold water, cover, and place on a low flame for 5–7 minutes. Let the grain or noodles slowly steam until hot and the vegetables are tender. Add tamari soy sauce, cover, and sauté for another 3–5 minutes. Place in serving bowls and garnish with chopped scallions, chives, or parsley.

Without Water. This method produces a drier, more separated grain or noodle dish. Brush a small amount of light or dark sesame oil in the bottom of a skillet and heat up. Add sliced vegetables and sauté for 1–2 minutes. Add the grain or noodles, mix in with the vegetables, and sauté for several minutes until the noodles or grains are hot and the vegetables are tender, but still slightly crisp. Season with a small amount of tamari soy sauce and cook for another 3–5 minutes over a medium to medium-high flame. In order for the moisture to evaporate, do not cover the skillet while cooking. When done, remove from the skillet, garnish, and serve.

BROWN RICE

Brown rice, now grown virtually around the world, is divided into three types. Short-grain rice is the smallest and hardiest of the three; it contains the most minerals and a high amount of gluten (the protein factor in grain). It is naturally sweet to the taste and the most suitable for consumption in temperate climates. Short-grain rice is especially delicious in breakfast porridge. Medium-grain rice is slightly larger and, when cooked, becomes softer and more moist than the other varieties. It, too, is excellent for regular consumption, especially in warmer regions. Long-grain rice, the longest variety, becomes very light and fluffy when cooked. It is prepared more often in tropical and semitropical areas, or during the hotter times of the year in temperate climates.

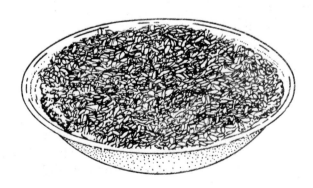

Pressure-Cooked Brown Rice

1 cup uncooked organic brown rice
1 1/2 cups water
Pinch of sea salt

Serves: 3–4

Place the washed rice in a pressure cooker and add the water. Place the cooker on a low flame, without covering and without adding the salt, for about 10 minutes or just until the water starts to boil. Next, add the sea salt and cover the cooker. Turn the flame up to high, and bring up to pressure. When the pressure is up, reduce the flame to medium-low, place a flame deflector under the cooker, and cook for 45–50 minutes. Next, remove the cooker from the flame and allow the pressure to come down. Remove the cover and let the rice sit for 4–5 minutes to loosen any grains on the bottom of the cooker. (This will make it easier for you to clean the pressure cooker and reduce any wasting of rice.)

To remove the rice from the cooker, take a wooden spoon or bamboo rice paddle, moisten it with cold water, and remove one spoonful of rice at a time from the cooker to a wooden bowl. Cover the bowl with a bamboo mat until ready to eat. This will prevent the rice from drying out.

For a different flavor, instead of using sea salt, try a 1-inch piece of kombu or a small umeboshi plum. Cook the same as above.

Boiled Brown Rice

1 cup uncooked organic brown rice
2 cups water
Pinch of salt

Serves: 3–4

Place the washed rice in a heavy stainless steel pot. Add the water and place on a low flame until the water starts to boil. Add the sea salt, cover, and reduce the flame to medium-low. Place a flame deflector under the pot and cook the rice for about 60 minutes. When done, remove from the flame and let sit for 4–5 minutes to loosen the rice on the bottom of the pot. Remove the rice and place in a wooden bowl.

Instead of using sea salt, try seasoning this dish with a small umeboshi plum or a 1-inch piece of kombu. Cook the same as above.

Soft Brown Rice (Rice Kayu)

1 cup uncooked organic brown rice
5 cups water
Pinch of sea salt, 1-inch strip of kombu, or 1 small umeboshi plum

Serves: 3–4

Place the washed rice in a pressure cooker. Add the water and one of the suggested seasonings. Cover the cooker, place on a high flame, and bring up to pressure. Reduce the flame to medium-low and cook for 45–50 minutes. Remove the cooker from the flame and allow the pressure to come down before removing the cover. Spoon the rice into individual serving bowls and garnish with a favorite condiment, strips of toasted nori, or chopped scallions. Serve while hot.

You can boil the rice instead of pressure cooking. Simply use the same measurements as above, but cook for 60 minutes. Serve as suggested.

Quick Brown Rice Porridge

1 cup cooked brown rice
3 cups water

Serves: 3–4

Place the cooked brown rice in a pot and add the water. Cover, place on a high flame, and bring to a boil. Reduce the flame to medium-low and simmer for 20–25 minutes or until the rice is soft and creamy. Serve same as above.

Soft Brown Rice and Winter Squash

1 cup uncooked organic brown rice
1 cup organic winter squash (buttercup, butternut, Hokkaido pumpkin,
red kuri, or gold nugget) cut into bite-sized chunks
5 cups water
Pinch of sea salt or 1-inch strip of kombu

Serves: 3–4

Place the washed rice and squash chunks in a pressure cooker or a heavy pot. Add water and one of the seasonings from the ingredient list. Cover and cook the same as for *Soft Brown Rice*, page 56.

For variation, try any of the following combinations of vegetables:

- Squash, cabbage, and carrots
- Carrots, cabbage, and onions
- Carrots, celery, and onions
- Daikon, shiitake mushrooms, and kombu
- Turnips and kombu

Simply wash the above vegetables, dice or cut into bite-sized chunks, and cook together with the rice as shown above.

Miso Soft Rice (Ojiya)

1 cup uncooked organic brown rice
5 cups water
1-inch strip kombu
3–4 scallion roots, finely chopped
3–4 scallion tops, thinly sliced
2 level teaspoons barley miso

Serves: 3–4

Place the washed rice, the kombu, and the water in a pressure cooker or heavy pot. Cook as directed for *Pressure-Cooked Brown Rice*, page 55 or *Boiled Brown Rice*, page 55. When the rice is done, remove from the flame. If pressure cooked, allow the pressure to come down. Remove the cover and place on a low flame. Add the sliced scallion tops to the cooked soft rice. Place the miso in a cup and add 2 teaspoons of cold water. Mix the miso and the water together and purée until smooth and creamy. Add the puréed miso and the scallion roots to the soft rice. Mix. Next cover the pot or pressure cooker (use a regular cover—do not pressure cook again) and let simmer without boiling for 2–3 minutes. Remove the cover and spoon rice into individual serving bowls. Serve while hot.

For a different flavor, try cooking the rice together with sliced daikon and shiitake mushrooms, then season with the miso and scallions.

Rice Balls (Musubi)

Water
2 cups cooked brown rice
1 umeboshi plum, halved
1 sheet nori, toasted and cut into 4 equal-sized pieces (see page 87 for instructions)

Yields: 2

Take a small bowl and fill it with cold water. Wet your hands slightly with the water. Take a handful of rice and form it into a round ball (as if making a snowball) or into a triangle by cupping your hands into a V-shape. Pack the rice firmly. Press a hole into the center and place half of the umeboshi plum inside. Pack the ball again to close the hole. Wet your fingers slightly and cover the rice ball or triangle with 2 pieces of nori, 1 piece at a time, so that it sticks to the rice. (See Figure 4.1.) You may have to wet your fingers occasionally to keep rice and nori from adhering to them, but be careful not to use too much water or the rice balls will lose some of their flavor. Repeat the above process with the remaining rice, nori, and umeboshi plum. You should now have 2 rice balls or triangles. Place on a platter and serve.

For a different flavor, instead of covering the rice balls with toasted nori, you can coat them with dry-roasted, ground sesame seeds; or roasted, chopped, and ground sunflower or pumpkin seeds. Simply wash, dry-roast, chop, and grind the seeds in a suribachi. After forming the rice balls, roll them in the ground seeds until completely coated.

Figure 4.1   Making a Rice Ball

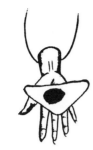

1. *Adding umeboshi plum.*

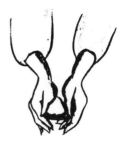

2. *Packing the rice ball.*

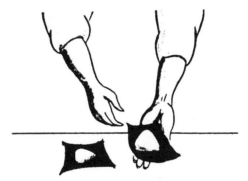

3. *Wrapping the rice ball with nori.*

Soft Rice and Raisins

1 cup uncooked organic brown rice
1/2 cup organic raisins
5 cups water
Pinch of sea salt

Serves: 3–4

Place the washed rice in a pressure cooker. Add the raisins, water, and sea salt. Cover, place on a high flame and bring up to pressure. Reduce the flame to medium-low and cook for 45–50 minutes. When done, remove from the flame and allow the pressure to come down. Remove the cover, spoon into individual serving dishes, and garnish with *Gomashio* (see page 152). Serve hot.

Instead of raisins, try using dried apples, pears, peaches, or apricots that have been soaked and sliced (the soaking water can be used as part of the water measurement).

Combination of Brown Rice and Grains

Brown rice, combined with other grains and cooked together, is very delicious. Some popular combinations are:

- 1/2 cup brown rice and 1/2 cup sweet brown rice
- 1/2 cup brown rice and 1/2 cup whole oats
- 1/2 cup brown rice and 1/2 cup millet
- 1/2 cup brown rice and 1/2 cup barley
- 1/2 cup brown rice and 1/2 cup hato mugi
- 1/2 cup brown rice and 1/3 cup millet and 1/3 cup whole oats
- 1/2 cup brown rice and 1 cup sweet corn

Simply wash the grain, add vegetables if desired, and cook with 5 cups of water as in *Soft Rice and Raisins*, page 59.

Vegetable and Tofu Fried Rice

1 tablespoon dark sesame oil
1/4 cup burdock, sliced into thin matchsticks
1/2 pound firm-style tofu, crumbled
1/4 cup carrots, diced
2 cups cooked brown rice
1/4 cup scallions, chopped
1–1 1/2 tablespoons tamari soy sauce

Serves: 3–4

Place the sesame oil in a skillet and heat up. Add the burdock and sauté for 1–2 minutes. Next, add the tofu, carrots, and cooked brown rice. Cover and reduce the flame to low. Simmer for 5–7 minutes. Add the scallions and tamari soy sauce, cover, and cook for another 3–5 minutes. Remove the cover, mix, and sauté 1–2 minutes longer. Remove and place in individual serving dishes. Serve while hot.

MILLET

Whole millet is the traditional staple of northern Asia and some parts of Europe and Africa. There are many varieties. Those grown in the United States and Canada are primarily yellow in color, while those in the Far East are often red. Because of its small, compact form, millet is rarely crushed or split. However, it may be ground into flour and used in baking. Much of the millet available in natural foods stores is organic in quality. Millet makes a deliciously sweet breakfast cereal, especially when cooked with naturally sweet vegetables.

Soft Millet with Miso (Millet Ojiya)

1 strip kombu, 1–2 inches long, soaked and diced
1/4 cup celery, sliced into 1/4-inch diagonals
1/2 cup daikon, cut into 1/2-inch-thick half-moons
1 cup winter squash (buttercup, butternut, Hokkaido pumpkin, gold nugget, red kuri, hubbard, acorn, delicata), cut into bite-sized pieces
1 cup uncooked organic millet
5 cups water
1/2 cup leeks, sliced into thin rounds
2 level teaspoons barley miso
Chopped parsley, chives, or scallions for garnish

Serves: 3–4

Place the kombu on the bottom of a heavy pot and put the celery on top of the kombu. Next, place the daikon on top of the celery. Layer the squash and millet on top of the daikon. Add the water, cover, and bring to a boil. Reduce the flame to medium-low and simmer for 30 minutes.

Reduce the flame to very low, so that the millet does not boil. Place the miso in a suribachi or bowl, add 3–4 teaspoons of water, and purée with a spoon or wooden pestle (surikogi). Wash the leeks and add to the millet and vegetables. Cover and simmer for 1–2 minutes. Next, add the miso, cover, and simmer for 2–3 minutes. Place in individual serving bowls, and garnish with chopped parsley, chives, or scallions.

Pressure-Cooked Millet

1 cup uncooked organic millet
5 cups water
Pinch of sea salt

Serves: 3–4

Place the washed millet in a pressure cooker along with the water and sea salt. Cover the cooker, place on a high flame, and bring up to pressure. Reduce the flame to medium-low and cook for 12–15 minutes. Remove from the flame and allow the pressure to come down. Remove the cover and spoon into individual serving dishes. Garnish with your favorite condiment and serve while hot.

   Instead of pressure cooking, bring the water to a boil in a heavy stainless steel pot, add the millet and sea salt, reduce the flame to medium-low, cover, and simmer for 30–35 minutes. Serve as above.

Soft Millet with Vegetables

1/4 cup onions, diced
1/2 cup cauliflower flowerets
1/4 cup cabbage, cut into 1-inch chunks
1 cup buttercup squash, cut into bite-sized chunks
1 cup uncooked organic millet
5 cups water
Pinch of sea salt

Serves: 3–4

Layer the vegetables in the following order in a heavy, stainless steel pot: onions, cauliflower, cabbage, and squash. Place the washed millet on top of the vegetables. Add the water and sea salt. Cover, bring to a boil, and then reduce the flame to medium-low. Simmer for 30–35 minutes until the vegetables and millet are very soft. Place in individual serving bowls, garnish with your favorite condiment, and serve while hot.

   Occasionally, for a quicker preparation, you may place all of the ingredients in a pressure cooker and cook for 15 minutes.

Millet Croquettes with Mushroom Sauce

3 cups cooked millet
1/2 cup onion, diced
1/4 cup parsley, chopped
1/4 cup whole wheat pastry flour
1/4 cup celery, thinly sliced
2 tablespoons dark sesame oil

Serves: 3–4

Mix all ingredients, except the sesame oil, together in a bowl. Take handfuls of the mixture, and form into balls. Then flatten out the balls to form 1/2-inch-thick patties or burgers. Heat up the oil in a skillet. Place the patties in the hot skillet and fry on both sides until golden brown. Remove to a serving dish.

MUSHROOM SAUCE

1 teaspoon light sesame oil
1/2 pound white mushrooms, thinly sliced
1/2 cup onion, diced
1/4 cup unbleached white or whole wheat pastry flour
2 cups water
Tamari soy sauce to taste

Heat the oil in a skillet, add the mushrooms, and sauté 1–2 minutes. Add the onions and sauté for another 2–3 minutes. Add the flour and mix in thoroughly with the vegetables. Slowly add the water, a little at a time, stirring constantly until the sauce is thick and smooth. Add several drops of tamari soy sauce for a mild salty taste. Pour the sauce over the millet croquettes and serve.

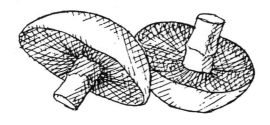

BARLEY AND PEARL BARLEY (HATO MUGI)

Barley has always been a traditional staple of ancient Egypt, Greece, Italy, and the Middle East. In the Far East there is a special type of whole barley called *pearl barley*, or hato mugi. Pearl barley is smaller, whiter, and more compact than ordinary barley. Especially delicious and soothing, pearl barley is traditionally used for medicinal and cosmetic purposes. There is also another type of barley called *pearled barley*, which is a milled form of the grain from which some vitamins and minerals have been removed. For ordinary, everyday use, unhulled or hulled organic whole barley is recommended. The different varieties of barley make wonderful breakfast porridges, especially when combined with short-grain brown rice.

Soft Barley Cereal

1 cup hulled barley
1 strip kombu, 1 1/2 inches long, soaked and diced (see page 87)
3 shiitake mushrooms, soaked, de-stemmed, and diced
1/2 cup carrots, diced
1/4 cup celery, diced
1/4 cup onion, diced
1/4 cup scallions, chopped
5 cups water

Serves: 3–4

Wash the barley, place in a bowl and cover with 4 cups water. Allow to soak for 6–8 hours or overnight. Place the barley and its soaking water in a pressure cooker. Add the kombu, shiitake mushrooms (along with their soaking waters), carrots, celery, and onions. Cover the cooker, place on a high flame, and bring up to pressure. Reduce the flame to medium-low and simmer for 50–60 minutes. Remove from the flame and allow the pressure to come down. Remove the cover from the cooker when all pressure is released. Place in individual serving bowls, garnish with chopped scallions and/or your favorite condiment.

Try using hato mugi (pearl barley) or Job's Tears instead of hulled barley. For a different flavor, you may season the cereal with a little puréed barley miso and simmer 2–3 minutes longer.

OATS

In antiquity, oats spread across northern Europe and became the principal food in Scotland, Ireland, and parts of England. Oats are now grown in many other parts of the world. Three forms are commonly available. Whole oats, from which only the outer husks have been removed, provide the most energy and vitality. They are preferred for everyday use, even though they take longer to prepare than the other two types. Scotch oats have been steamed and steel-cut into small pieces. They create a very chewy dish. Rolled oats have been steamed and passed through rollers. Although the most common form of oatmeal eaten today, rolled oats retain less energy and nutrients than whole oats. Still, they may be prepared from time to time and are often the best quality grain available while traveling or eating out. Oats are also puffed, processed into flakes, and ground into flour for baking.

Pressure-Cooked Whole Oats

1 cup whole oats, dry-roasted (see page 50)
5 cups water
Pinch of sea salt

Serves: 3–4

Place all ingredients in a pressure cooker, cover, and soak overnight. In the morning, place on a high flame and bring up to pressure. Reduce the flame to medium-low and cook for 50–60 minutes. Remove from flame, allow the pressure to come down, and remove the cover. Spoon into serving bowls and garnish with your favorite condiment, a few raisins, or a little brown rice syrup. Serve hot.

Boiled Whole Oats

1 cup whole oats
4–5 cups water
Pinch of sea salt

Serves: 3–4

Wash the oats, place in a strainer, rinse, and allow to drain. Heat up a skillet and place the damp oats in. Dry-roast the oats until they are slightly golden and they release a nutty fragrance. Place the roasted oats in a heavy stainless steel pot and add the water and sea salt. Cover the pot and bring to a boil. Reduce the flame to low and simmer, stirring occasionally, several hours.

For a sweeter flavor, try cooking the oats with 1/2 cup organic raisins. The oats can also be sweetened with a spoonful of rice syrup drizzled over each serving. Plain oats are also delicious with a little *Gomashio* (page 152) sprinkled on top.

Rolled Oat Cereal (Oatmeal)

1 cup rolled oats, dry-roasted (see page 50 for roasting instructions)
2–3 cups water
Pinch of sea salt

Serves: 3–4

Place the roasted oats in a heavy pot and add the water and sea salt. Cover and bring to a boil. Reduce the flame to low and simmer for 20–25 minutes. Place in serving bowls, garnish, and serve.

Try cooking the oats together with 1/2 cup of diced or thinly sliced onions. Occasionally, 1/4 cup of raisins may be cooked together with the oats for a sweeter flavor.

Steel-Cut Oats (Irish or Scotch Oats)

1 cup steel-cut oats
2–2 1//2 cups water
Pinch of sea salt

Serves: 3–4

Place the water in a saucepan and bring to a boil. Add the oats and sea salt, cover, and reduce the flame to low. Simmer for 25–30 minutes. Place in individual serving bowls, garnish, and serve.

SWEET BROWN RICE

Sweet brown rice is more glutenous than regular brown rice and is also slightly sweeter to the taste. It is primarily used in making mochi, amazake, cookies, crackers, and other special foods. Mochi is delicious in the morning when eaten with hot miso soup.

Soft Sweet Brown Rice Cereal

1 cup uncooked sweet brown rice
5 cups water
Pinch of sea salt

Serves: 3–4

Place all of the ingredients in a pressure cooker or heavy pot and cook in the same manner as for *Soft Brown Rice (Rice Kayu)*, page 56.

Sweet Rice Mochi

Mochi (pounded sweet rice dumplings) can be bought prepackaged in most macrobiotic and natural foods stores. It is hard and cut into small squares. The mochi puffs up and becomes soft and digestible when cooked. You can also make your own deliciously sweet mochi at home. It is fun, can involve your family and friends, and is quite inexpensive.

2 cups uncooked organic sweet brown rice
2–2 1/2 cups water
Pinch of sea salt per cup of rice

Serves: 3–4

In a bowl, cover the washed rice with water and allow to soak 6–8 minutes or overnight. Place the rice, soaking water, and sea salt in a pressure cooker. Cover, place over a high flame, and bring up to pressure. When the pressure is up, reduce the flame to medium-low, and place a flame deflector under the cooker. Cook for 45–50 minutes. Remove from the flame and allow the pressure to come down. Remove the cover and let sit for 4–5 minutes to loosen the bottom grains of rice from the cooker. Remove the cooked rice and place it in a thick wooden bowl. Take a heavy wooden pestle or mochi pounder and moisten it under cold water. Pound the sweet rice vigorously for approximately 45–60 minutes, or until the grains are completely crushed and become very sticky.

Take a standard-sized baking sheet and coat it with brown rice flour. Spread the pounded sweet rice evenly on the baking sheet. Now, cover the sheet with a thin layer of cotton cheesecloth and let sit for 1–2 days until the mochi is hard and dry. When ready, slice the mochi into 2-inch squares, wrap in wax paper or a paper bag, and refrigerate until ready to use.

For variety, try pounding in 1/2 cup of soaked raisins with the sweet rice to produce raisin-mochi, which is a sweet and very delicious treat. Instead of raisins, or in combination with raisins, try adding roasted sesame or sunflower seeds to the sweet rice and pound. There are many types of mochi you can make: sweet brown rice and millet; sweet brown rice and mugwort; sweet brown rice and soaked, dry-roasted Japanese black soybeans.

Sesame-Mochi Cakes

1/2 cup sesame seeds
1 cup uncooked organic sweet rice
1–1 1/4 cups water
Pinch of sea salt

Serves: 3–4

Wash, soak, and cook the rice as in *Sweet Rice Mochi* (page 67). Pound the sweet rice for 20–30 minutes.

Wash the sesame seeds, the same as you would grains (page 44), place in a strainer, and drain. Place the damp sesame seeds into a hot, stainless steel skillet. Dry-roast over a high flame until most of the moisture has evaporated from the seeds, then reduce the flame to medium-low. Dry-roast, stirring constantly with a wooden rice paddle until the seeds begin to puff up and pop. The best way of testing whether the seeds are completely roasted is to fill a tablespoon with the toasted seeds, then pour them back into the skillet. If the seeds stick to the tablespoon, they still contain moisture, and should be toasted longer. If no seeds stick to the tablespoon, the seeds are done. Quickly remove the seeds, as they will quickly burn if left in the hot skillet. Place the roasted seeds in a suriba-chi. You can either leave the seeds whole, or take a wooden pestle and grind the seeds to a fine powder (about 80 percent crushed).

Next, take 1 heaping tablespoon of freshly pounded mochi, and place it into the suribachi with either the whole roasted sesame seeds or the ground sesame-seed powder. Roll the pounded mochi in the seeds until completely coated. Pick up the coated mochi and form it into a ball. Now, flatten the ball in the palm of your hand to form a small sesame-coated cake. Repeat with the remaining mixture. Eat as is or with a little grated daikon and a drop or two of tamari soy sauce.

Toasted Mochi

Several 2-inch squares of mochi

Heat up a stainless steel or cast iron skillet over a medium flame. Place the mochi squares in the hot skillet so that they do not touch each other. Cover the skillet, then reduce the flame to low, and cook until slightly browned. Turn the squares over and brown the other side. The mochi is ready when it is slightly puffed and lightly browned. Remove the cooked mochi and place on individual plates. Serve with a little grated daikon and a couple drops of tamari soy sauce on each square.

You may also toast a sheet of nori (page 87) and cut it into 1 x 4-inch strips. Then wrap a strip around each piece of mochi before serving with grated daikon and tamari soy sauce.

Sweet Mochi with Kinako
(Roasted Soybean Flour)

1/4–1/3 cup brown rice syrup
1/2 cup roasted soybean flour (kinako)
Several pieces mochi

Toast the mochi as instructed in *Toasted Mochi* (above). Place the rice syrup in a saucepan and bring to a boil. Remove from the flame. Dip the toasted mochi in the sweet rice syrup. Remove and roll the sweetened pieces of mochi in the roasted soybean flour (kinako) until completely coated. Remove and place on a serving platter.

WHOLE CORN AND CORN PRODUCTS

Native Indian corn, or maize, has been grown for millenia in South, Central, and North America. The original varieties of corn were smaller, more compact, and hardier than the larger hybrid varieties that have replaced them. Native American and Latin American corn cuisine was based primarily on the use of masa, or whole corn dough. Masa is made from corn kernels taken from the cob, dried, cooked with wood ashes and water, and used as the basis for making tacos, tostadas, arepas, empanadas, and other traditional corn dishes. These whole grain preparations retain the basic energy and vitality of the whole corn. Today, however, many of the corn dishes in Mexican restaurants or those available in supermarkets are made with refined cornmeal and artificial ingredients rather than the whole corn dough and other natural foods.

Most modern corn dishes are prepared with cornmeal, the flour made from whole corn. Though retaining lesser energy and nutrients than corn dough, good quality, organic, unrefined cornmeal that does not have any chemicals, sugar, or other refined or artificial ingredients may be used from time to time to make breakfast cereal, corn bread, corn muffins, and other corn dishes. A coarsely ground form of cornmeal is corn grits, a popular warm breakfast cereal in the southern United States. A crispy, flaky form of cornmeal, popular as a cold breakfast food in the northern United States, is corn flakes. Naturally processed corn flakes or puffed whole corn are used on occasion in macrobiotic breakfasts and can be eaten with amazake or rice milk, instead of cow's milk.

Corn Grits

1 cup white or yellow corn grits
3 cups water
Pinch of sea salt

Serves: 3–4

Place the water and sea salt in a heavy stainless steel pot and bring to a boil. In a strainer, quickly wash the corn grits and then place into the boiling water. Cover and bring to a boil again. Reduce the flame to medium-low and simmer for 20–30 minutes, stirring occasionally. Place in individual serving dishes. Garnish with your favorite condiment, a few raisins, or a little brown rice syrup, and serve while hot.

Polenta (Cornmeal)

1 cup cornmeal
3 cups water
Pinch of sea salt

Serves: 3–4

Place water in a saucepan and bring to a boil. Add the sea salt. Slowly pour the cornmeal into the boiling water, stirring constantly to prevent lumping. Bring to a boil again, stirring constantly until thickened. Reduce the flame to medium-low and simmer, covered, for 35–40 minutes. Remove from the flame and place in individual serving bowls. Garnish and serve.

Fried Polenta

1 cup cornmeal
3 cups water
Pinch of sea salt
Dark sesame oil
Tamari soy sauce

Serves: 3–4

Cook the cornmeal as instructed in the recipe for *Polenta* (above). When done, pour the thick cereal into a glass bread pan or baking dish. Set aside and allow to cool completely. When hard, slice the polenta into 1 × 3-inch pieces.

Brush a skillet with sesame oil and heat up. Fry the polenta several minutes on both sides until golden brown. While frying, you may sprinkle 1–2 drops of tamari soy sauce on each side for a slightly salty flavor. Remove and place on a serving platter. These polenta slices can be served plain or with a small amount of grated daikon.

For variety, try adding some fresh sweet corn or chopped onions to the cornmeal while boiling. Cook until done. Allow to cool, slice, and fry as above. For a sweeter flavor, you can pour a little heated, sweet rice syrup or barley malt over the fried polenta.

Arepas

Arepas are traditional corn cakes from South America, made from whole, dried, cooked corn. Pure wood ashes are initially cooked together with the whole corn to soften the hard outer shells. Then the corn is rinsed to remove the wood ash, and cooked again in plain water. The cooked corn is then ground in a flour mill producing a corn dough called masa. The masa is then formed into cakes and pan-fried or baked to produce a delicious corn cake, which is much easier to digest than whole corn. Arepas are delicious treats at breakfast or anytime.

2 cups whole dry flint corn
10 cups water, divided in half
1 cup pure, sifted wood ash
1/8 teaspoon sea salt
Dark sesame oil
Cheesecloth

Yield: Approximately 8–10

Wash the whole corn and place in a bowl. Add 5 cups of water to cover the corn. Soak for 6–8 hours or overnight. Place the corn and soaking water in a pressure cooker. Tie the pure wood ash up in cheesecloth so that it cannot fall out and place in a pressure cooker. Place the cover on the cooker, bring up to pressure over a high flame, reduce the flame to medium-low, and cook for about 45–60 minutes. Remove from the burner and allow the pressure to come down. Take the cover off the cooker and discard the cheesecloth sack. Pour the corn into a bowl and wash to remove any wood ash from the corn. Place in a colander, rinse with cold water, and drain.

To make the masa, place the partially cooked corn (no wood ash remaining) into a clean pressure cooker. Cover and bring up to pressure. Reduce the flame to medium-low and cook for 60 minutes. Remove from the flame and allow the pressure to come down before removing the cover. Place the corn in a steel flour mill and grind in a bowl. Knead the masa for about 15–20 minutes by hand. After kneading, add the sea salt and a small amount of water to form a dough the consistency of bread dough. Form the dough into several tennis-sized balls. Then press the balls with the palms of your hands to form 1/2 inch-thick patties or round cakes. Bring a pot of water to a boil and place the cakes in. Boil and remove when the cakes rise to the surface.

Brush a cast iron skillet with sesame oil and heat up. Place the corn cakes in the hot skillet, cover, and pan-fry each side for 2–4 minutes or until a crust forms on the cakes. Remove the cakes, place on an oiled baking sheet, and bake for about 20 minutes at 350° F. When done, the arepas will puff up slightly and will produce a hollow thumping sound when tapped with your fingers.

Arepas may be eaten plain, with a tamari soy sauce dip, or with a little naturally made jam or jelly spread on top. For variety, try slitting the arepas open when they are done cooking, and stuff them with cooked vegetables. For a delicious treat, mix grated or diced onion, roasted sesame seeds, or finely chopped vegetables into the masa before pan-frying and baking.

BUCKWHEAT

The traditional staple of Russia, Eastern Europe, and parts of central and northern Asia, buckwheat is the hardiest of the cereal plants because of the cold weather it endures. Its kernels are called groats, and are usually roasted and eaten in their whole form or in coarse or fine granules. All of these forms of buckwheat are known as kasha. Whenever available, the whole groats should be used, as they retain more energy and nutrients than the granules. In the Far East, buckwheat is used primarily in making noodles, or soba, while in the West, the deep rich taste of buckwheat flour is often enjoyed in pancakes and waffles.

Creamy Buckwheat Cereal

5 cups water
Pinch of sea salt
1 cup dry-roasted buckwheat groats (see page 50 for roasting instructions)
2 tablespoons chopped scallions or parsley for garnish

Serves: 3–4

Put the water and sea salt in a saucepan and bring to a boil. Place the dry-roasted buckwheat into the pan, cover, reduce the flame to medium-low, and simmer for 20–30 minutes. When done, place the chopped scallions or parsley in the hot cereal, stir, and serve.

For variety, add diced onions, celery, carrots, or cabbage to the buckwheat from the beginning of cooking.

Buckwheat Dumplings

1 cup buckwheat flour
Pinch of sea salt
2 cups cold water
1/2 teaspoon fresh ginger, grated
2 tablespoons scallions, finely chopped
1/2 sheet nori, toasted and cut into bite-sized pieces (see page 87)

Yield: Approximately 12

Bring a pot of water to a boil. In a mixing bowl, mix the flour, sea salt, and water together to produce a batter. Take a heaping tablespoon of batter and drop it into the boiling water. You can cook a few dumplings at a time, but be careful not to crowd them or they will stick together. Cook until they rise to the surface of the water. Remove, drain, and place 2–3 dumplings in individual serving bowls. Garnish each serving with a dab of grated ginger, a few chopped scallions, and several pieces of toasted nori.

Quick and Creamy Buckwheat Cereal (Sobagaki) with Dashi

2 cups dry-roasted buckwheat flour (see page 50 for roasting instructions)
2 cups boiling water
Pinch of sea salt
1/2 teaspoon fresh ginger, grated
2 tablespoons scallions, finely chopped
1/2 sheet nori, toasted and cut into bite-sized pieces (see page 87)

DASHI (Kombu Broth)

2 cups water
1 strip kombu, 3–4 inches long
1 tablespoon tamari soy sauce

In a heated skillet, pour the boiling water over the roasted flour. Mix vigorously for 2–3 minutes or until the water is completely absorbed. Mix in the sea salt and cook over a medium flame for another 3–4 minutes.

To prepare the dashi, put the water and kombu strip in a saucepan, cover, and bring to a boil. Reduce the flame to low and simmer for 3–4 minutes. Remove the kombu and set aside for future use. Season the dashi with tamari soy sauce, reduce the flame to low, and simmer another 3–5 minutes.

To serve the creamy buckwheat cereal, spoon into individual serving bowls. Spoon a little dashi over each serving and garnish with a dab of freshly grated ginger, a few chopped scallions, and several pieces of the toasted nori.

WHOLE WHEAT AND WHEAT PRODUCTS

In its whole form, wheat is difficult to digest unless it is chewed very well. It is also best if soaked several hours or overnight, as it takes longer to cook than other grains, and is more easily digested if soaked prior to cooking. Wheat is usually cracked, partially processed, or milled into flour for breads and pastas. These partially processed foods are easier to prepare, chew, and digest than whole wheat. However, whole wheat can be combined with other grains to make delicious morning cereals.

Whole Wheat and Brown Rice Cereal

1/4 cup whole wheat berries
1 cup uncooked organic brown rice
5 cups water
Pinch of sea salt

Serves: 3–4

Wash the wheat berries and rice separately, then place them together in a bowl. Cover with the water and allow to soak for 6–8 hours or overnight. Place in a pressure cooker with the soaking water and sea salt. Cover the cooker, place over a high flame, and bring up to pressure. Reduce the flame to medium-low and cook for 60 minutes. Remove from the flame and allow the pressure to come down. Remove the cover, place in serving bowls, garnish, and serve.

Bulgur and Vegetables

2 1/2–3 cups water
Pinch of sea salt
1 cup bulgur
1/4 cup onion, diced
1/4 cup carrot, diced
1/4 cup cabbage, diced
1 teaspoon celery leaves, chopped

Serves: 3–4

Place the water and sea salt in a pot and bring to a boil. Add the vegetables and the bulgur. Cover, bring to a boil again, reduce the flame to medium-low, and simmer for about 20 minutes. Remove, place in serving bowls, garnish, and serve.

Simple Boiled Fu

1/2 package (1.75 ounces) round fu, soaked
and sliced into bite-sized pieces
2 cups water
2–3 teaspoons tamari soy sauce
2 tablespoons scallions, chopped
1/2 teaspoon fresh ginger, grated

Serves: 3–4

Place the fu and water in a saucepan. Cover, bring to a boil, reduce the flame to medium-low, and simmer for about 10 minutes. Add the tamari soy sauce, cover, and simmer for another 5 minutes. Add the grated ginger and simmer 1 more minute. Remove from the flame and place in individual serving bowls. Garnish with chopped scallions and serve.

Homemade Seitan

3 1/2 pounds whole wheat bread flour
7–8 cups cold water
6–7 cups warm water
1 strip kombu, 3 inches long
3–4 slices fresh ginger, 1/8 inch thick
1/4–1/3 cup tamari soy sauce

Serves: 3–4

Place the flour in a large mixing bowl. Gradually, add part of the cold water, mixing it together with the flour until it is the consistency of bread dough. Knead the dough for about 5–10 minutes. Leave the kneaded dough in the bowl and cover it with the warm water. Let the dough sit in the warm water for 10–15 minutes.

Knead the dough again while it is in the bowl of soaking water. The water will become cloudy and milky. Pour off the cloudy water into a large jar (save this cloudy starch water). Add the remainder of cold water to cover the dough and gently knead again. Pour off the starch water into the jar again. Repeat once more, saving the starch water. Place the gluten in a colander, kneading it again under alternating streams of cold and warm water, until most of the bran is washed out of the gluten. The cloudy starch water that was reserved can be used as a thickening agent for stews, gravies, and sauces, or if allowed to sit for 3–4 days and becomes sour, it can be used as a sourdough starter for breads, waffles (see *Sourdough Waffles*, page 168), and pancakes.

After the bran and starch are washed from the gluten, it will form a sticky ball. Place 6–7 cups of water in a pot and bring to a boil. Drop the whole ball of gluten into the boiling water, or separate it into 5 or 6 smaller balls. Cook for about 5 minutes or until the balls float. Remove the ball or balls and slice into 1/4–1/2-inch-thick pieces. Place the kombu, ginger slices, tamari soy sauce, and sliced gluten pieces into the pot of boiling water. Cover and bring to a boil again. Reduce the flame to medium-low and simmer for 35–45 minutes. The seitan is now ready to use.

To store, remove the kombu and discard. Pour the salty tamari soy sauce cooking liquid into a jar along with the cooked slices of seitan. Allow to cool. Cover and refrigerate until ready to use.

Seitan and Fu

Whole wheat seitan and fu are both high-protein products made from wheat gluten. They are both commonly used as meat substitutes in macrobiotic cooking.

Seitan, sometimes referred to as "wheat meat," is a gluten product that has been simmered in a mixture of tamari soy sauce, water, and kombu. Although a little more difficult to digest than noodles or fu, its rich flavor and rough texture can be enjoyed, on occasion, at breakfast. Seitan can be purchased in most macrobiotic and natural foods stores, usually prepackaged in eight- or sixteen-ounce packages. This prepackaged, ready-to-eat seitan can simply be sliced and eaten as is, or heated up by pan-frying, steaming, baking, boiling, or broiling. If you have the time and feel creative, try the recipe for *Homemade Seitan* on page 77, which is very delicious. You can make enough for several days, as seitan will keep in the refrigerator for about one week. Simply store in a tightly sealed container.

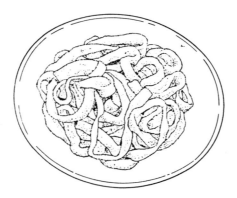

Fu is made in the same manner as seitan, but instead of boiling the gluten in water and tamari soy sauce, it is lightly toasted in a hot oven, steamed, sliced, and allowed to dry out completely. After drying, it is wrapped or sealed in airtight containers. Fu is available in several forms: flat sheets, thick large rounds, or small rounds. Fu made from 100 percent whole wheat flour is the best quality. Like noodles and pasta, fu is easy to digest. It can be used in breakfast soups or vegetable dishes. To reconsititute dried fu, simply place in a bowl, cover with warm water, and let soak for about 7–10 minutes until soft. Remove from the soaking water, squeeze out any excess, and slice the rounds into bite-sized pieces, or cut the fu into thin, flat noodles or 1-inch squares.

Whole Wheat Fu and Vegetables

1/2 cup onion wedges
1/2 cup carrots, cut into diagonals
1/2 package (1.75 ounces) round fu, soaked
and sliced into bite-sized pieces
2 cups water (include fu soaking water)
1 cup broccoli flowerets
2 teaspoons tamari soy sauce
Chopped scallions for garnish

Serves: 3–4

Place the onions, carrots, fu, and water in a pot. Cover, bring to a boil, reduce the flame to medium-low, and cook for about 5 minutes. Add the broccoli, cover, and simmer for another 2–3 minutes. Add the tamari soy sauce and simmer an additional 2–3 minutes. Remove and place in individual serving bowls, garnish with a few chopped scallions, and serve.

Pan-Fried Seitan

1 cup cooked seitan slices (see *Homemade Seitan* recipe, page 77)
Dark sesame oil

Brush a small amount of oil on a skillet or pancake griddle and heat up. Place the seitan slices on the hot skillet and pan-fry each side for 2–4 minutes or until slightly browned. The slices may be eaten as is or garnished with a little grated daikon. Pan-fried seitan also makes delicious sandwiches.

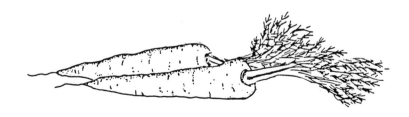

Pan-Fried Udon, Pasta, or Soba

2 quarts water
1 package udon, soba, or your favorite pasta (8 ounces)
Dark or light sesame oil
1/2 cup onions, sliced into thin half-moons
1/2 cup carrots, sliced into matchsticks
1/4 cup celery, sliced into thin diagonals
1/2 cup Chinese cabbage, sliced into 1-inch squares
Tamari soy sauce

Serves: 3–4

Place the water in a pot, cover, and bring to a boil. (If you are cooking whole wheat pasta or spaghetti, place a small pinch of sea salt in the water. Japanese udon and soba contain salt and are best cooked in unsalted water.) Place the udon, soba, or pasta in the boiling water. Stir, do not cover, and bring to a boil again. Simmer several minutes until the noodles are tender. To test for doneness, take a noodle and break it in half. If it is done, the noodle will be the same color inside and out. If not done, the outside will be dark, while the inside of the noodle will be white. When the noodles are done, pour them into a strainer or colander and rinse with cold water until completely cool. Let sit and drain for several minutes.

Brush a skillet with a little sesame oil and heat up. Sauté the onions for 1–2 minutes. Next, add the carrots and celery and sauté for another 1–2 minutes. Place the Chinese cabbage in the skillet and sauté several seconds. Place the drained udon, soba, or pasta on top of the vegetables. Cover the skillet, reduce the flame to low, and simmer for several minutes until the vegetables are done and the noodles are hot. Add several drops of tamari soy sauce, and cook for another 3–4 minutes. Mix the noodles and vegetables together, remove, and place in a large serving bowl.

RYE

Whole rye, like wheat, is a little difficult to digest in its whole form unless chewed very well. It is usually milled into flour for making bread. However, you can soak rye overnight and combine it with other grains to make a soft morning cereal.

Soft Rye and Brown Rice Cereal

1/4 cup organic whole rye
1 cup uncooked organic brown rice
5 cups water
Pinch of sea salt

Serves: 3–4

Wash the rye and brown rice, place in a bowl, and add the water. Soak the rye and rice 6–8 hours or overnight. Place the rye, rice, soaking water, and the sea salt in a pressure cooker. Cover and place over a high flame. Bring up to pressure, reduce the flame to medium-low, and simmer for 60 minutes. Remove from the flame and allow the pressure to come down before removing the cover. Place cereal in individual serving bowls, garnish, and serve.

AMARANTH, QUINOA, AND TEFF

In addition to the grains already mentioned, a variety of other wild and domestic cereal grains are used in macrobiotic breakfasts. These include amaranth, the traditional grain of the Aztec civilization; quinoa, the staple of the ancient Incan Empire; and teff, a staple grain of Ethiopia and other parts of Africa. These grains can be used in making delicious and nourishing breakfast porridges.

Amaranth Morning Cereal

3 cups water
Pinch of sea salt
1 cup amaranth, washed, rinsed, and drained

Serves: 3–4

Place the water and sea salt in a pot, cover, and bring to a boil. Add the amaranth, cover, and reduce the flame to medium-low. Simmer for 20–25 minutes. Place in individual serving bowls and serve hot. For a sweeter taste, add some raisins or other soaked, chopped, and dried fruit to the amaranth while cooking.

Boiled Quinoa

2 cups water
Pinch of sea salt
1/4 cup raisins
1/2 cup quinoa, washed, rinsed, and drained

Serves: 3–4

Place the water, sea salt, and raisins in a pot. Cover and bring to a boil. Stir in the quinoa, cover, and bring to a boil again. Reduce the flame to medium-low and simmer for 10 minutes. Turn off the flame and let sit for 5 minutes. Place in individual serving dishes.

Teff Porridge

Pinch of sea salt
2 cups water
1/2 cup teff, washed, rinsed, and drained

Serves: 3–4

Place the sea salt and water in a pot, cover, and bring to a boil. Add the teff, cover, and bring to a boil again. Reduce the flame to medium-low and simmer for 15–20 minutes. Remove and place in individual serving dishes.

Chapter Five

MISO AND OTHER BREAKFAST SOUPS

Soups are not a separate category of food as much as a way of cooking and combining foods. They are especially easy to digest in the morning. Digestion is the process of breaking down foods into a liquid medium. By allowing foods to cook in broth, we accelerate this process. The notion that soups are easy to digest is a part of folk tradition around the world. They are often the first foods served to someone who is ill. Soup is usually eaten at the beginning of the meal to ease the stomach and digestive organs into functioning, although you don't need to finish it before starting to eat your other dishes. Although we don't usually think of soup as a breakfast food, miso soup has been used at breakfast for centuries in the Far East. It is especially delicious when served with a whole grain porridge and other simple side dishes.

MISO SOUP

Miso is a dark purée made from soybeans, unrefined sea salt, and fermented barley or rice. Natural miso contains living enzymes that aid digestion and strengthen the quality of the blood. This wholesome food provides a nutritious balance of complex carbohydrates, essential oils, protein, vitamins, and minerals. It is traditionally prepared by allowing the ingredients to ferment slowly in wooden kegs. Miso is used, both in macrobiotic and traditional cooking, as a base for soups as well as a seasoning for other dishes.

Natural miso is gaining recognition as an important food in a healthful way of eating. In 1981 the National Cancer Center of Japan announced the results of a ten-year study on the effects of miso soup on health. They discovered that people who ate miso soup daily were less likely to develop heart disease, digestive cancers, and liver disease. The best miso is naturally aged for several summers or longer and is made from whole, round soybeans—without chemically treated ingredients or artificial aging procedures. It has a deep, rich flavor. Barley (mugi) miso is normally the best for regular use at breakfast, followed by soybean (hatcho) miso. Other misos, most of which are aged for less time than these varieties, can be used on occasion. Quickly aged misos are often saltier than the mild-tasting, longer-aged barley miso.

Diluting Miso

Approximately 1/2–1 teaspoon of miso is used per cup of liquid. Because miso is a thick and sometimes chunky purée, it needs to be diluted before being added to soup. This helps it dissolve more thoroughly and blend into the broth. To dilute miso, place it in a suribachi or a bowl and add a small amount of hot broth or plain water. Purée the miso with a wooden pestle (surikogi), or mix thoroughly with a spoon. It is now ready to add to your broth.

Cooking Miso

Miso contains living enzymes that aid digestion and strengthen the digestive organs. Boiling miso can inhibit the beneficial activity of these enzymes. In most cases, therefore, we suggest that you simply allow miso to simmer for several minutes rather than boiling it. Uncooked miso has a somewhat harsh flavor and a tightening effect on the body, and is not recommended. If you are using miso as a seasoning and not necessarily for its beneficial enzymes, then you may occasionally boil it over a low flame for several minutes after adding it to soup.

Preparation Methods for Miso Soup

There are many ways to prepare miso soup in the morning. Although morning miso soup is best kept simple and light, stronger, richer soups can also be enjoyed on occasion, especially during cold weather. Below are the most commonly used methods for preparing miso soup.

Method One: With Boiling Water

This method is used most often in making miso soup. The vegetables cook more quickly and the flavor is very light and delicate.

First, place water in a pot, cover, and bring to a boil. Wash, soak, and slice any sea vegetables you will be using and add them to the boiling water. Cover the pot, bring the water to a boil again, and reduce the flame to medium-low. Simmer the sea vegetables for 2–3 minutes. Next, add any sliced land vegetables you will be using, cover, bring to a boil again, and reduce the flame to medium-low. Simmer the vegetables for 5–7 minutes or until tender. Reduce the flame to very low, so that the water does not boil. Place miso in a bowl or suribachi, add a small amount of hot soup broth or plain water, and purée the miso until smooth. Spoon the puréed miso into the hot water and let it simmer for 2–3 minutes. Your soup is now ready to be garnished and served.

Method Two: With Cold Water

This method produces a richer, heartier soup in which the vegetables become very tender and nearly melt in your mouth. Place sliced land and sea vegetables in a pot and add your cold water measurement. Cover the pot, place on a high flame, and bring to a boil. Reduce the flame to medium-low and simmer for 10–15 minutes until the vegetables are very soft and tender. Reduce the flame to very low, add the puréed miso, and simmer for 2–3 minutes before garnishing and serving.

Method Three: With Layered Ingredients

This method produces soup with a very sweet flavor and a peaceful, calming energy. Layer your ingredients in a pot, with the vegetables on the bottom and any grains or beans on the top. Any style of cutting may be used, as long as the vegetables are sliced so that they are about the same thickness for uniform cooking. Then, add water to almost cover the top of the vegetables. Cover the pot, place on a high flame, and bring to a boil. Reduce the flame to medium-low and simmer several minutes until the vegetables are tender. Being careful not to disturb the layered ingredients, slowly add more water until the desired consistency is produced. Cover, bring to a boil, reduce the flame to medium-low, and let the soup cook for several more minutes. Reduce the flame to very low, add puréed miso, and simmer for 2–3 minutes. Mix the ingredients just before garnishing and serve.

Method Four: With Sautéed Vegetables

This method also produces a very rich and hearty soup. Although we don't recommend using oil on a regular basis at breakfast, you can use it on occasion. Vegetables can be sautéed in water or in a small amount of

Using Sea Vegetables in Miso Soup

Sea vegetables are included among the most nutritious foods. For centuries they have been valued for their health-giving and disease-preventing properties. Dried sea vegetables are rich in complex carbohydrates, fiber, protein, vitamins, and minerals, and they are low in fat. Plants from the sea contain, proportionally, more minerals than any other type of food. Nori, for instance, has from two to four times more vitamin A than carrots and ten times more than spinach. Hijiki, wakame, and arame have from eleven to fourteen times more calcium than milk. Kombu, wakame, arame, hijiki, and nori have from three to eight times more iron than meat. Sea vegetables are also a major source of iodine. If they are included regularly, refined, chemically iodized salt is not necessary. They are also proportionally higher in vitamin A, thiamine, riboflavin, vitamin B_6, vitamin B_{12}, and niacin than most land vegetables and fruits. Nori is also rich in vitamin C and protein. Sea vegetables are especially delicious when eaten in morning miso or other soups.

Practically all of the ingredients in traditional miso soup are associated with lower risk of disease. As we have seen, miso itself is associated with a lower incidence of cancer and heart disease. Recent studies have also shown that sea vegetables lower cancer risk and inhibit the development of tumors. Orange-yellow vegetables, such as carrots and squash, and leafy green vegetables are used often in miso soup. These vegetables are high in beta carotene, a compound that has also been shown to reduce cancer risk. For more information on the preventive value of these and other foods used in the macrobiotic diet, please see our book *The Macrobiotic Cancer Prevention Cookbook* (Avery, 1988).

Below, the sea vegetables most commonly used in soups are discussed. Additional information on cutting methods for sea vegetables can be found on page 88.

- **Wakame** has a very light, delicate texture and a moderately salty taste. It is the most frequently used sea vegetable in miso soup. It cooks quickly, and the soaking water from wakame can sometimes be added to the broth. If the soaking water is very salty, it is best diluted before being used.

  To prepare wakame for use in soup, place it in a bowl and cover with cold water. Swish it around with your hands, pour the water off, and repeat twice. Put the wakame in a strainer, rinse quickly under cold water, and place in a bowl. Cover with cold water and soak for 3–5 minutes until it is soft enough to slice. Taste the soaking water. If it is overly salty, dilute it with plain water. Discard if it is very salty.

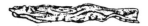

Kombu

Wakame

- **Kombu** has a very mild, salty flavor. If you are planning to eat the kombu, it requires 30–35 minutes to cook. If you are using it to flavor the soup stock, it needs to be simmered for only 3–5 minutes. It can also be saved and used to flavor other dishes. The soaking water is almost always used.

  To prepare kombu, first wipe it with a clean, damp sponge. It should then be soaked and sliced in the same manner as wakame (see above).

- **Nori** has a very mild flavor. Since it tends to fall apart when boiled, it is usually not cooked in soup, but used as a garnish.

  Sheet nori does not require washing or soaking, but is roasted by rotating it several inches above a gas flame until its color changes from black to dark green. (This process only takes a few seconds.) You can see the change in color easily by holding the sheet up to a light or window. Once toasted, the sheet can be folded into halves or quarters and used in such recipes as *Rice Balls (Musubi)*, found on page 58, or it can be broken up into bite-sized pieces for garnishing soups.

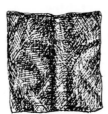

Nori sheet

- **Dulse** has a fairly salty flavor and becomes milder after being soaked. The soaking water is often too salty for use in soup stock. Use the same soaking method for dulse that is used in preparing wakame (see above).

high quality sesame oil. To water sauté, add enough water to just cover the bottom of the pot. Sauté the vegetables with the strongest flavors first and then the milder-flavored ones; for example, onions first, then celery, cabbage, and finally carrots. To oil sauté, brush a small amount of light or dark sesame oil on the bottom of the pot and heat up. Sauté as above.

When the vegetables are finished sautéing, add them, along with the desired amount of water, to a pot. Cover, place on a high flame, and bring to a boil. Reduce the flame to medium-low and simmer for several minutes until the vegetables are tender. Reduce the flame to very low, add the puréed miso, then simmer for 2–3 minutes. Garnish and serve.

How Cutting Methods Influence Taste

How we cut our vegetables greatly influences the flavor and energy of our soups. Let us see what the effects are from the most commonly used methods of cutting.

Very Thin or Diced.   These methods leave a great deal of exposed surface in each slice, which permits additional flavor and nutrients to readily diffuse throughout the broth. They produce a flavorful broth and milder-tasting vegetables. Thinly sliced vegetables cook much more quickly than larger slices and add a lighter, more diffused energy to soups.

Thick Slices or Chunks.   Larger cuts produce less exposed surface in each piece, thus giving the broth a milder flavor. However, the vegetables tend to retain more distinct flavor and nutrients. Larger slices or chunks take longer to cook than smaller slices; they impart a calm, peaceful energy to soup.

Cutting Methods for Sea Vegetables

Sea vegetables can be cut in basically the same way that other vegetables are cut. However, as we have seen, with the exception of nori, they are usually soaked prior to being cut, which makes them soft and slippery. They need to be handled a little differently from land vegetables, which are more firm and solid.

When slicing wakame, spread the soaked sea vegetable on a cutting board as you would a leafy green vegetable. Cut away the hard stem, as with leafy greens, and slice finely. Stack the leafy portions on top of each other and slice straight across or on the diagonal.

To slice kombu, spread it on the cutting board and slice into 1-inch squares or $2 \times 1/2$-inch rectangles.

Soaked dulse, arame, or hijiki can simply be placed on the cutting board and sliced thinly or thickly on the diagonal.

Soaking Other Ingredients

Other dried foods, such as dried tofu, shiitake mushrooms, fu (dried wheat gluten), dried daikon, and occasionally yuba (dried soymilk curd), are also used in miso soup. With the exception of dried shredded daikon, these foods do not require washing. Dried daikon can simply be quickly washed and rinsed before being added to soup. Table 5.1 presents guidelines for soaking dried foods.

Garnishing Soups

Garnishes help balance the taste, energy, and color of breakfast soups. Thinly sliced raw scallions, for example, add fresh light energy to miso and other soups. Miso soup has a rich brown color that looks much more appealing when garnished with chopped scallions, chives, watercress, celery, or other bright green vegetables.

Using Leftover Vegetables

Leftover vegetables can also be used in miso soup. First, prepare the soup stock, season with miso, and then add the leftover vegetables while the soup is still simmering. Leftovers don't need to be boiled (a simple reheating will do). Overcooking them detracts from their flavor, color, and nutritional content. When storing leftovers, place them in the refrigerator or in a cool pantry. It is a good idea to use them as quickly as possible. Cooked vegetables and other foods lose flavor and nutrients if they are kept for too long.

Table 5.1   Guidelines for Soaking Dried Foods

Food	Water Temperature	Water Quantity	Soaking Time (minutes)	Use for Water
Dried tofu	Warm	Cover	5–7	Discard
Fu	Warm	Cover	5–7	Use
Shiitake	Warm	Cover	10–15	Use
Dried daikon	Cold	Cover	3–5	Use if light-colored
Dried burdock	Warm	Cover	10–15	Use
Dried lotus	Warm	Cover	30–40	Use
Yuba	Warm	Cover	5–7	Discard

Preparing Broth Ahead of Time

You can also use pre-made broth to make breakfast soup. At dinner, set aside unseasoned broth for use the following morning. Place the appropriate amount of unseasoned broth in a tightly sealed jar and refrigerate. In the morning, remove the broth, place it in a saucepan, and bring to a boil. Purée about 1/2 teaspoon of miso for each cup of broth. Reduce the flame to very low and add the diluted miso. Cover and simmer for 2–3 minutes. Place in serving bowls and garnish. This method is preferable to simply reheating leftover soup from the night before.

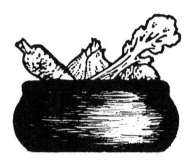

Basic Miso Soup

4–5 cups water
1/4–1/2 cup dry wakame (1/2–1 ounce), soaked and sliced into
1/4–1/2-inch pieces (see inset on page 86)
1–1 1/2 cup onions, sliced into thin half-moons
1 1/2–2 1/2 tablespoons puréed barley miso
Chopped scallions for garnish

Yield: 4–5 cup servings

Place the water in a pot, cover, and bring it to a boil. Add the sliced wakame and soaking water (if it is not salty), cover, and bring to a boil again. Reduce the flame to medium and simmer for about 2–3 minutes. Add the onions, cover, and simmer another 5–7 minutes or until the onions and wakame are tender. Reduce the flame to very low, so that the water does not boil.

Dilute the miso with a few tablespoons of the broth and add to the pot. Cover and simmer for 2–3 minutes. Place in individual serving bowls, garnish each bowl with a few chopped scallions, and serve while hot.

Onion-Carrot-Tofu Miso Soup

4–5 cups water
1/4 cup dry wakame (1/2 ounce), soaked and sliced
(see inset on page 86)
1/2 cup onions, sliced into thin half-moons
1/2 cup carrots, sliced into thin matchsticks
1/2 cup firm-style tofu (1/3 pound), cut into 1/4 × 1/2-inch cubes
1 1/2–2 1/2 tablespoons puréed miso
Chopped scallions for garnish

Yield: 4–5 cup servings

Place the water in a pot, cover, and bring to a boil. Add the wakame, bring to a boil again, reduce the flame to medium, and simmer for 2–3 minutes. Next add the onions, cover, and simmer for 1–2 minutes. Add the carrots, cover, and simmer for 4–5 minutes until the vegetables are tender. Reduce the flame to very low. Add the tofu to the soup. Dilute the miso with a few tablespoons of the broth and add to the pot. Cover and simmer for 2–3 minutes. Place in individual serving bowls, garnish with a sprinkling of chopped scallions, and serve.

Daikon-Wakame Miso Soup

4–5 cups water
1/4 cup dry wakame (1/2 ounce), soaked and sliced
(see inset on page 86)
1 cup daikon, sliced into thin rounds, half-moons, quarters, or rectangles
1 1/2–2 1/2 tablespoons puréed miso
Chopped scallions for garnish

Yield: 4–5 cup servings

Place the water in a pot, cover, and bring to a boil. Add the wakame, cover, and reduce the flame to medium. Simmer for 2–3 minutes. Add the daikon, cover, and simmer for another 5 minutes. Reduce the flame to very low, so that the soup does not boil. Dilute the miso with a few tablespoons of broth and add it to the pot. Cover and simmer for 2–3 minutes. Place in individual serving bowls and garnish with chopped scallions.

Daikon-Shiitake Miso Soup

4–5 cups water
3–4 shiitake mushrooms, soaked, de-stemmed, and finely sliced
1/4 cup dry wakame (1/2 ounce), soaked and sliced
(see inset on page 86)
1 cup daikon, sliced into thin rounds or half-moons
1 1/2–2 1/2 tablespoons puréed miso
Chopped scallions, chives, parsley, or celery for garnish

Yield: 4–5 cup servings

Place the water in a pot, cover, and bring to a boil. Add the shiitake to the boiling water, cover, and reduce the flame to medium. Put the sliced wakame into the boiling water, cover, and simmer for 2–3 minutes. Add the daikon, cover, and simmer for another 3–5 minutes, depending on the thickness of the daikon. Reduce the flame to very low. Dilute the miso with 2–3 tablespoons of the broth, add it to the soup, and simmer for another 2–3 minutes. Remove, place in serving bowls, garnish, and serve.

Quick Cup of Miso Soup

1 cup water
1 tablespoon carrots, cut into thin matchsticks
1/8–1/4 cup scallions, chives, parsley, or celery leaves, sliced
1/2–1 teaspoon puréed miso
1/2 sheet nori, toasted and cut into 1-inch squares
(see page 87)

Yield: 1 cup serving

Place the water in a pot, cover, and bring to a boil. Add the carrots, cover, and simmer 45 seconds. Reduce the flame to very low. Dilute the miso with a few tablespoons of the broth and add to the soup along with the scallions. Simmer for 2–3 minutes. Place in a serving bowl and garnish with several pieces of toasted nori.

Miso Soup with Sweet Rice Dumplings

4–5 cups water
1/4 cup dry wakame (1/2 ounce), soaked and sliced
(see inset on page 86)
1 cup daikon root, sliced into thin rounds, half-moons, or rectangles
1 cup daikon greens, cut into 1/2-inch lengths
1 1/2–2 1/2 tablespoons puréed miso
Chopped scallions for garnish

Yield: 4–5 cup servings

SWEET RICE DUMPLINGS

1/2 cup sweet rice flour or brown rice flour
1/4 cup boiling water
Small pinch of sea salt (optional)

Yield: 10–12 dumplings

Place the water in a pot, cover, and bring to a boil. Add the wakame, cover, reduce the flame to medium-low, and simmer for 2–3 minutes. Add the daikon root, cover, and simmer for 3–4 minutes or until tender.

While the daikon is cooking, place the sweet rice flour and pinch of sea salt into a small bowl. Add the boiling water to the sweet rice flour and mix with your hands. Take a teaspoon of the flour mixture in your hands and form it into a round ball. With your thumb, make a thumbprint into the ball. The ball should resemble a small cake or dumpling now. Repeat until several dumplings have been made and the dough is used up.

When the daikon is cooked, drop the dumplings into the soup broth along with the daikon greens. Simmer covered until the dumplings float to the surface of the broth. Reduce the flame to very low. Dilute the miso with a few tablespoons of the broth and add it to the soup. Simmer for 2–3 minutes. Garnish with chopped scallions, parsley, or chives.

Try any of the following combinations for delicious miso soup: daikon, shiitake, and sweet rice dumplings; daikon, celery, shiitake, and sweet rice dumplings; celery, shiitake, and sweet rice dumplings; daikon, taro potato, shiitake, celery, and sweet rice dumplings.

French Onion Miso Soup

Although this soup is served mainly as part of an evening meal with roasted or pan-fried croutons for garnish, we have adjusted it for breakfast by including vegetables such as peas, green beans, or corn, and have omitted the croutons. It can be served on a cool fall or winter morning or when you feel the need to have a little extra oil in your diet. If you wish, you can omit the oil sautéing, and simply water-sauté the onions. Then cook as directed.

Dark sesame oil
2 cups onions, thinly sliced into half-moons
3 shiitake mushrooms, soaked and thinly sliced
1 strip kombu, 3–4 inches long, soaked and sliced into very thin strips
(see inset on page 87)
4–5 cups water
1/2 cup green peas, green beans, or sweet corn
1 1/2–2 1/2 tablespoons puréed miso
Chopped parsley for garnish

Yield: 4–5 cup servings

Place a small amount of sesame oil in a pot and heat up. Add the onions and sauté for 2–3 minutes. Next, add the shiitake and kombu. Add the water (including the soaking waters from the shiitake and the kombu). Cover, bring to a boil, reduce the flame to medium-low, and simmer for about 15–20 minutes until the onions, shiitake, and kombu are tender. Add the green peas, cover, and simmer for 4–5 minutes until tender, but still bright green. Reduce the flame to very low. Dilute the miso with a little broth from the pot, add it to the soup stock, cover, and simmer for 2–3 minutes. Place in individual serving bowls and garnish.

Miso Soup with Squash Skins

Did you ever wonder what to do with leftover, uncooked skin from winter squash such as buttercup, butternut, Hokkaido pumpkin, red kuri, or gold nugget? Quite often, when preparing puréed squash soups, removing the skins is recommended to keep the color of the soup a nice yellow-orange, instead of green. These mineral and vitamin-rich (if unwaxed) skins can be used in preparing morning miso soup, which makes it deliciously sweet.

4–5 cups water
1/4 cup dry wakame (1/2 ounce), soaked and sliced
(see inset on page 86)
2 cups uncooked winter squash skins, sliced into thin matchsticks
1/2 cup leeks, sliced into very thin rounds
1 1/2–2 1/2 tablespoons puréed miso
Chopped scallions, chives, or parsley for garnish

Yield: 4–5 cup servings

Place the water in a pot, cover, and bring to a boil. Add the wakame, cover, reduce the flame to medium-low, and simmer for 2–3 minutes. Next, add the squash skins and leeks, cover, and simmer 4–5 minutes. Reduce the flame under the soup pot to very low. Dilute the miso with a few tablespoons of the broth and add to the soup. Cover and simmer 2–3 minutes. Place in serving bowls, garnish, and serve.

Natto Miso Soup

4–5 cups water
1/4 cup wakame (1/2 ounce), soaked and sliced
(see inset on page 86)
2 cups celery, sliced into thin diagonals
1 1/2–2 1/2 tablespoons puréed miso
1/2 cup natto
Chopped scallions, chives, or parsley for garnish

Yield: 4–5 cup servings

Place the water in a pot, cover, and bring to a boil. Place the wakame in the boiling water, cover, reduce the flame to medium-low, and simmer for about 2–3 minutes. Add the celery, cover, and simmer for 3–5 minutes until the celery is tender. Dilute the miso with a few tablespoons of the broth and add it to the soup. Cover and simmer for 2–3 minutes. Place the natto in the soup and simmer for about a minute. Place in serving bowls, garnish, and serve.

Okara Miso Soup

Okara is a by-product of the tofu-making process. It is a great source of protein, nutrients, and fiber.

4–5 cups water
1 strip kombu, 4 inches long, soaked and sliced into thin matchsticks
(see inset on page 87)
1/2 cup fresh or dried daikon, soaked and cut into 1/2-inch lengths
2 shiitake mushrooms, soaked, de-stemmed, and thinly sliced
1/2 teaspoon dark sesame oil (optional)
1/2 cup fresh okara
1/4 cup burdock, shaved or thinly sliced
1/4 cup carrots, sliced into matchsticks
1 1/2–2 1/2 tablespoons puréed miso
Chopped scallions, parsley, or chives for garnish

Yield: 4–5 cup servings

Place the water (including the soaking waters from the kombu, dried daikon, and shiitake) in a pot, cover, and bring to a boil. Add the prepared daikon, kombu, and shiitake. Bring to a boil again, reduce the flame to medium-low, and simmer about 25–30 minutes until the daikon and kombu are tender.

While the vegetables are simmering, heat the dark sesame oil in a skillet, add the okara, and sauté for 4–5 minutes, stirring often to prevent scorching. Add the burdock to the soup after the other vegetables have cooked for about 15–20 minutes. Cover and simmer for another 5–7 minutes. Add the carrots and okara. Simmer for 2–3 minutes, then reduce the flame to very low. Dilute the miso with a few tablespoons of the broth and add to the soup. Cover and simmer for 2–3 minutes. Remove, place in serving bowls, and garnish.

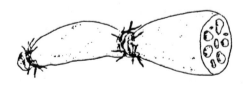

Lotus root

Oyster Mushroom and Leek Miso Soup

4–5 cups water
1 strip kombu, 3–4 inches long, soaked and sliced into thin matchsticks
(see inset on page 87)
1 cup leeks, sliced into 1/4-inch rounds
1/2 cup carrots, sliced into thin matchsticks
1 cup oyster mushrooms, sliced
1 1/2–2 1/2 tablespoons puréed barley miso
1/2 pound fresh firm-style tofu, cubed
Chopped parsley for garnish

Yield: 4–5 cup servings

Place the water in a pot, cover, and bring to a boil. Place the kombu and the soaking water in the pot, cover, and bring to a boil again. Simmer over a medium-low flame for about 20 minutes. After the kombu has cooked for 20 minutes, add the leeks and carrots. Cover and simmer for 3–5 minutes. Add the oyster mushrooms and simmer for 2–3 minutes. Reduce the flame to very low. Dilute the miso with a few tablespoons of the broth and add it to the soup along with the tofu cubes. Simmer for 2–3 minutes. Remove, place in individual serving bowls, garnish, and serve.

Miso Soup with Lotus Root Dumplings

4–5 cups water
1 strip kombu (3–4 inches long)
1 1/2–2 1/2 tablespoons puréed miso
Several small sprigs fresh watercress for garnish

Yield: 4–5 cup servings

LOTUS ROOT DUMPLINGS

1/4 cup whole wheat pastry flour
1/3–1/2 cup lotus root, finely grated
1–2 tablespoons boiling water

Yield: 10–12 dumplings

Place the water and kombu in a pot, cover, and bring to a boil. Reduce the flame to medium-low and simmer for about 4–5 minutes. Remove the kombu and set aside to be used later in other dishes.

While the water is coming to a boil and the kombu is cooking, mix the whole wheat pastry flour, the lotus root, and 1–2 tablespoons of water together in a small bowl. Mix thoroughly. Take a teaspoonful of the lotus mixture and roll it into a small ball with your hands. Repeat until the mixture is used up and you have several lotus root balls. When the kombu is finished cooking and has been removed from the pot, place the balls, one at a time, into the boiling water. When the dumplings rise to the surface of the water, they are done.

Reduce the flame to very low. Dilute the miso with a few tablespoons of the broth and add it to the soup. Simmer for 2–3 minutes. Place several small sprigs of washed watercress in each individual serving bowl. Next, ladle the soup and 1 or 2 dumplings into each bowl. The hot miso soup will be sufficient to cook the watercress. Serve while hot.

Green Peas and Fu Miso Soup

1 cup fu, soaked and sliced into bite-sized rounds
4–5 cups water
2 cups fresh green peas, shelled
1 1/2–2 1/2 tablespoons puréed miso
1 sheet nori, toasted and cut into thin strips (see page 87)
Chopped chives for garnish

Yield: 4–5 cup servings

Place the fu and 4 cups water (include the fu soaking water as part of your measurement) in a pot. Cover, bring to a boil, reduce the flame to medium-low, and simmer for about 10 minutes until the fu is soft. Place 1 cup of water in a saucepan and bring to a boil. Place the peas in the saucepan, cover, and simmer for 4–5 minutes until tender, but still bright green in color. Remove the peas and drain in a colander. Make sure to save the cooking water and add it to the soup with the fu. Reduce the flame to very low. Dilute the miso with a few tablespoons of the broth and add it, along with the peas, to the soup. Simmer for 2–3 minutes. Place the soup in individual serving bowls, garnish with several strips of toasted nori and a sprinkle of chopped chives.

For variety, instead of green peas, try fresh green or yellow waxed beans, fresh sweet corn, carrot matchsticks, or lima beans.

Carrot, Burdock, and Dulse Miso Soup

4–5 cups water
1/4 cup burdock, shaved
1/4 cup carrots, sliced into matchsticks
1/4 cup dry dulse (1/2 ounce), soaked and sliced (see inset on page 87)
1/4 cup kale, cut into 1-inch squares
1 1/2–2 1/2 tablespoons puréed miso
Chopped scallions for garnish

Yield: 4–5 cup servings

Place the water in a pot, cover, and bring to a boil. Place the burdock in the boiling water, cover, and simmer for 3–4 minutes. Add the carrots and dulse, cover, and simmer for 4–5 minutes or until the burdock is tender. Add the kale, cover, and simmer for 1–2 minutes. Reduce the flame to very low. Dilute the miso with a few tablespoons of the broth and add it to the soup. Cover and simmer for 2–3 minutes. Remove, place in serving bowls, and garnish with a few chopped scallions.

Fresh Shiitake Mushroom Miso Soup

4–5 cups water
1/4 cup dry wakame (1/2 ounce), soaked and sliced
(see inset on page 86)
5–6 fresh shiitake mushrooms, de-stemmed and quartered
1 tablespoon bonita flakes (optional)
1/2 cup snow peas, de-stemmed
1/2 cup firm-style tofu (4 ounces), cut into 1-inch cubes
1 1/2–2 1/2 tablespoons puréed miso

Yield: 4–5 cup servings

Place the water in a pot, cover, and bring to a boil. Add the wakame, cover, reduce the flame to medium-low, and simmer for 2–3 minutes. Add the shiitake mushrooms and the bonita flakes to the soup. Cover and simmer for 4–5 minutes. Place the snow peas and the tofu in the pot. Reduce the flame to very low. Dilute the miso with a few tablespoons of the broth and add it to the soup. Cover and simmer for 2–3 minutes. Remove and place in serving bowls.

Celery and Tofu Miso Soup

4–5 cups water
1/4 cup dry wakame (1/2 ounce) soaked and sliced
(see inset on page 86)
1/4 cup onions, sliced into thin half-moons
1/2 cup celery, sliced into thin diagonals
1 cup firm-style tofu (8 ounces), cut into 1-inch cubes
1 1/2–2 1/2 tablespoons puréed miso
Chopped parsley for garnish

Yield: 4–5 cup servings

Place the water in a pot, cover, and bring to a boil. Place the wakame in the boiling water, cover, reduce the flame to medium-low, and simmer for 2–3 minutes. Add the onions and celery, cover, and simmer for 4–5 minutes or until tender. Add the tofu cubes. Reduce the flame to very low. Dilute the miso with a few tablespoons of the broth and add to the pot. Cover and simmer for 2–3 minutes. Place in serving bowls and garnish with chopped parsley.

Mochi Miso Soup

8–10 pieces of mochi, 1 × 2 inches (see recipe on page 67)
4–5 cups water
1 cup Chinese cabbage leaves, sliced into 1/2-inch diagonals
1 1/2–2 1/2 tablespoons puréed miso
1 sheet nori, toasted and cut into strips or squares(see page 87)
Chopped scallions for garnish

Yield: 4–5 cup servings

Place the pieces of mochi into a heated skillet. Cover, reduce the flame to low, and pan-fry until slightly browned. Turn the mochi pieces over, cover, and brown the other side. When done, both sides of the mochi should be browned and the pieces should be slightly puffed. Remove and place 1 or 2 pieces of the pan-fried mochi in each serving bowl.

Place the water in a pot, cover, and bring to a boil. Add the Chinese cabbage, cover, reduce the flame to medium-low, and simmer for 1–2 minutes. Reduce the flame to very low. Dilute the miso with a few tablespoons of the broth and add it to the soup. Cover and simmer for 2–3 minutes. Pour the hot soup over the mochi slices in the serving bowls. Garnish each bowl of soup with several pieces of toasted nori and a few chopped scallions.

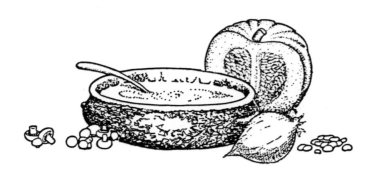

Squash and Cabbage Miso Soup

4–5 cups water
1/4 cup dry wakame (1/2 ounce), soaked and sliced
(see inset on page 86)
1/4 cup onions, sliced into thin half-moons
1 cup buttercup, gold nugget, red kuri squash, or Hokkaido pumpkin,
cut into 1-inch squares or chunks
1 cup green cabbage, cut into 1-inch squares
1 1/2–2 1/2 tablespoons puréed miso
Chopped scallions, chives, or parsley for garnish

Yield: 4–5 cup servings

Put the water in a pot, cover, and bring to a boil. Place the wakame in the boiling water, cover, and reduce the flame to medium-low. Simmer for 2–3 minutes. Add the onions, squash, and cabbage. Cover and simmer for 5–7 minutes until the vegetables are tender. Reduce the flame to very low. Dilute the miso with a little broth from the pot and add to the soup. Simmer for 2–3 minutes. Remove, place in serving bowls, and garnish with chopped scallions, chives, or parsley.

Watercress and Carrot Miso Soup

4–5 cups water
1 strip kombu, 3–4 inches long, soaked
1/2 cup carrots, cut into thin diagonals
1 1/2–2 1/2 tablespoons puréed miso
1 cup watercress sprigs (1/2 bunch)
Chopped scallions for garnish

Yield: 4–5 cup servings

Put the water in a pot along with the kombu (and its soaking water). Cover and bring to a boil. Reduce the flame to medium-low and simmer for 3–4 minutes. Remove the kombu and set aside for later use in other dishes. Add the carrots, cover, and simmer for 1–2 minutes. Reduce the flame to very low. Dilute the miso with a little broth from the pot and add to the soup. Cover and simmer for another 2–3 minutes. Place 1 or 2 sprigs of watercress in each serving bowl. Ladle the hot miso soup over the watercress. Let sit several seconds, garnish with scallions, and serve.

Noodle or Pasta Miso Soup

4–5 cups water
3–4 shiitake mushrooms, soaked and sliced
1/4 cup dry wakame (1/2 ounce), soaked and sliced
(see inset on page 86)
1/2 cup onions, sliced into thin half-moons
1/4 cup celery, sliced into thin diagonals
1 1/2–2 1/2 tablespoons puréed miso
8 ounces cooked udon, somen, or pasta (leftovers can be used)
1/4 cup scallions, chopped

Yield: 4–5 cup servings

Place the water in a pot, cover, and bring to a boil. Add the shiitake, cover, and simmer for 5–7 minutes. Add the wakame, cover, and simmer for 3–4 minutes. Add the onions and celery, cover, reduce the flame to medium-low, and simmer for 4–5 minutes or until tender.

Reduce the flame to very low. Dilute the miso with a little broth from the pot and add to the soup along with the cooked noodles or pasta. Simmer for 2–3 minutes. Add the scallions, mix, and place in serving bowls.

Brown Rice and Scallion Miso Soup

4–5 cups water
1/4 cup dry wakame (1/2 ounce), soaked and sliced
(see inset on page 86)
1 tablespoon scallion roots, minced
2 cups cooked brown rice (leftovers can be used)
1 1/2–2 1/2 tablespoons puréed miso
1 cup scallion tops, sliced

Yield: 4–5 cup servings

Place the water in a pot, cover, and bring to a boil. Add the wakame, cover, reduce the flame to medium-low, and simmer for 2–3 minutes. Add the scallion roots and the brown rice. Cover and simmer for 7–10 minutes. Reduce the flame to very low. Dilute the miso with a little broth from the pot and add to the soup along with the scallion tops. Cover and simmer for 2–3 minutes. Remove and place in serving bowls.

Millet and Squash Miso Soup

4–5 cups water
1 cup cooked millet (leftovers can be used)
1/4 cup onions, diced
1/4 cup celery, diced
1 cup buttercup, butternut, gold nugget, red kuri squash, or
Hokkaido pumpkin, cut into 1-inch chunks
1 1/2–2 1/2 tablespoons puréed miso
1 sheet nori, toasted and cut into bite-sized pieces (see page 87)
Chopped parsley for garnish

Yield: 4–5 cup servings

Place the water in a pot, cover, and bring it to a boil. Add the millet, onions, celery, and squash. Cover, reduce the flame to medium-low, and simmer for about 10 minutes. Reduce the flame to very low. Dilute the miso with a little broth from the pot and add to the soup. Cover and simmer for 2–3 minutes. Ladle the hot soup into serving bowls and garnish with several pieces of toasted nori and some chopped parsley.

OTHER SOUP STOCKS

Although miso is a popular base for morning soups, there are other commonly used soups, as well. Listed below are some of these soup stocks and how to prepare them. Soups made from these stocks are generally prepared in the same manner as recipes using miso as their base.

Kombu Stock

Take a 3-inch piece of kombu, dust it off, and soak for 3–5 minutes. Place the kombu and soaking water in a pot. Add about 4 cups of fresh water, cover, and bring to a boil. Reduce the flame to medium-low and simmer for 3–4 minutes. Remove the kombu and set aside for use in other dishes. The unseasoned stock can now be seasoned with tamari soy sauce, or can be cooked with vegetables before any seasoning is added.

Shiitake Mushroom Stock

Place 2–3 dried shiitake mushrooms in a small amount of warm water to cover. Soak for about 10 minutes. Remove, squeeze out liquid, and remove the very bottom portion of the hard, woody stem with a vegetable knife. Place the shiitake (either whole or sliced) in a pot and add 4 cups of fresh water plus the water used to soak the shiitake. Cover and bring to a boil. Reduce the flame to medium-low and simmer for about 10 minutes. If you choose not to use the shiitake in the soup, remove and set aside for use in other dishes. The stock is now ready to be seasoned with tamari soy sauce. You can cook your vegetables in it before adding the tamari.

Kombu-Shiitake Stock

Soak the kombu and shiitake and place them in a pot along with their soaking waters. Add 4 cups fresh water, cover, and bring to a boil.

Reduce the flame to medium-low and simmer for 3–4 minutes. Remove the kombu and set aside. Cover again and simmer the shiitake for another 5–7 minutes. Remove the shiitake and set aside for future use. The stock is now ready.

Vegetable Stock

These stocks can be made from naturally sweet vegetables such as carrots, onions, squash, and cabbage, or from unused ends or pieces of vegetables. Commonly used odds and ends include the tops and root tips of carrots or other root vegetables, scallion roots, cabbage cores, corn cobs or husks, pea pods, the tough outer leaves of cabbage or cauliflower, squash skins, and celery leaves. Generally, we don't use vegetable pieces that have strong, bitter flavors such as burdock root, carrot greens, and watercress, as these tend to overpower the soup.

To prepare, simply place the vegetable pieces in a pot with 4–5 cups of water. Cover and bring to a boil. Reduce the flame to medium-low and simmer for 5 minutes (for a milder stock) or for 10 minutes (for a stronger stock). The stock is now ready to use.

SEASONING SOUPS

Cooking with Tamari Soy Sauce

Natural soy sauce is known in macrobiotics as tamari. We recommend using only the highest-quality soy sauce made from organically grown soybeans and wheat, good-quality water, and unrefined sea salt. The ingredients are combined and the soy sauce is allowed to age naturally for several years in well-aged cedar vats. Modern, commercial soy sauces are far different products. They are made with defatted soybean meal, chemically grown grains, and refined salt; they usually contain monosodium glutamate, caramel, sugar, and other additives or preservatives. They are aged artificially in temperature-controlled, stainless steel or epoxy-coated vats, which reduces their aging process considerably. Where natural soy sauce is aged for years, commercial brands are only aged for several months, at best. Their taste is also harsh and flat in comparison to natural tamari soy sauce.

In most cases, tamari soy sauce is added to the broth after the other ingredients have almost finished cooking and is then simmered over a low flame for about 5–7 minutes. This allows the sea salt contained in the tamari to thoroughly penetrate the vegetables and other ingredients. Boiling the stock after the tamari has been added may cause the sea salt to be poorly absorbed and can give your soup a bitter taste. Soups are much more flavorful when the tamari is simply simmered.

Cooking with Sea Salt

The quantity of salt, the amount consumed, and the way salt is used in cooking are all important issues in creating a healthful diet. In proper volume, high-quality, unrefined, natural sea salt, containing trace minerals, contributes to good overall health. Traditionally processed, unrefined sea salt, usually available only in natural foods stores or through mail-order companies, contains compounds of several minerals such as magnesium, as well as trace amounts of about sixty other elements commonly found in the sea. The proportion of trace minerals varies according to the way the salt is processed, usually from a high of about 3 percent to a low of about 0.5 percent.

There are various types of sea salt, ranging in color from white, to off-white, to gray. White sea salt is the best for daily use. Gray or off-white salt is not recommended for cooking, but can be used when making pickles that require a long time for aging.

Regular table salt is a highly refined product consisting of about 99.5 percent sodium chloride. While it is made from either sea salt or rock salt, most of the natural trace elements have been removed due to processing. Dextrose, a highly refined industrial sugar, is customarily added to table salt to stabilize the iodine and to make the crystals stick to foods.

When you use sea salt to flavor soups or stocks, add a very small pinch at the beginning to bring out the natural sweetness of the vegetables and grains. The remaining sea salt can be added toward the end of cooking. Once salt has been added, let the soup cook for 10–15 minutes. This will give the salt a chance to thoroughly dissolve and be absorbed by the ingredients. This also gives the salt a less harsh quality and enhances the natural sweetness of the ingredients in the soup.

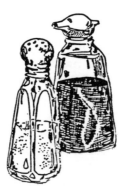

Simple Rice and Scallion Soup

4–5 cups kombu or kombu-shiitake soup stock (see page 104)
2 cups cooked brown rice (can use leftovers)
2–3 tablespoons tamari soy sauce
1 cup scallions, thinly sliced
1 sheet nori, toasted and cut into bite-sized strips or squares
(see page 87)
1/2 teaspoons ginger juice (optional)

Yield: 4–5 cup servings

Place soup stock in a pot, cover, and bring to a boil. Add the brown rice, cover, reduce the flame to medium-low, and simmer for about 5 minutes. Season with the tamari soy sauce and simmer another 5 minutes. Place in serving bowls. Garnish each bowl with 2–3 tablespoons of the sliced scallions, several pieces of toasted nori, and a drop or two of fresh ginger juice.

Unseasoned Clear Soup

1/2 cup carrots, sliced into thin matchsticks
1 bunch watercress, sliced into 1-inch lengths
4–5 cups kombu or kombu-shiitake soup stock (see page 104)
1 cup firm-style tofu (8 ounces), cut into 1-inch cubes
1 sheet nori, toasted and cut into bite-sized strips or squares
(see page 87)
1/2 teaspoon ginger juice
Chopped scallions for garnish

Yield: 4–5 cup servings

In a saucepan, bring a small amount of water to a boil. Place the carrots in the water, cover, and boil 1–2 minutes. Remove the carrots and drain. In the same saucepan, place the watercress, cover, and simmer for 45 seconds. Remove, rinse under cold water, and drain.

In a pot, bring the soup stock to a boil. Add the tofu, reduce the flame to low, and simmer for 1–2 minutes or until it floats. (Tofu that is overcooked becomes hard and rubbery, making it more difficult to digest.) Place several pieces of cooked carrots and watercress in individual serving bowls. Pour the hot kombu stock and tofu over the carrots and watercress. Garnish each bowl of soup with several pieces of toasted nori and a drop or two of freshly grated ginger juice. Top with a sprinkling of chopped scallions and serve.

Noodles and Vegetables in
Tamari Soy Sauce Broth

4–5 cups kombu or kombu-shiitake soup stock (see page 104)
1/2 cup carrots, sliced into thin matchsticks
1 cup Chinese cabbage, sliced into 1-inch squares
2–3 tablespoons tamari soy sauce
8 ounces cooked udon, somen noodles, or other pasta
(leftovers can be used)
1/4 cup scallions, thinly sliced
1 sheet nori, toasted and cut into bite-sized strips or squares
(see page 87)

Yield: 4–5 cup servings.

Place the stock in a pot, cover, and bring to a boil. Add the carrots and cabbage to the hot soup stock. Cover, bring to a boil, reduce the flame to low, and simmer for 1–2 minutes. Season with tamari soy sauce and simmer another 4–5 minutes. Place cooked udon, somen noodles, or other pasta in individual serving bowls. Pour the hot tamari soy sauce broth and vegetables over the noodles. Garnish with sliced scallions and several pieces of toasted nori.

Mochi Soup

8–10 pieces toasted mochi (see recipe on page 67)
4–5 cups boiling water or light bancha tea (see page 162)
1 sheet nori, toasted and cut into bite-sized strips or squares
(see page 87)
Several drops of tamari soy sauce
1/4 cup scallions, sliced
Yield: 4–5 cup servings

Place 1–2 pieces of toasted mochi in each individual soup bowl. Pour boiling water or bancha tea over the mochi. Garnish with several pieces of toasted nori and 2–3 drops of tamari soy sauce for each serving. Top with a sprinkling of sliced scallions.

Corn Soup

4–5 cups water
1/2 cup white or yellow corn grits, uncooked
2 cups fresh sweet corn
1/8 teaspoon sea salt
1 sheet nori, toasted and cut into bite-sized strips or squares
(see page 87)
Chopped parsley for garnish

Yield: 4–5 cup servings

Place the water in a pot, cover, and bring to a boil. Slowly add the corn grits, stirring constantly to prevent lumping. Add the sweet corn, cover, and reduce the flame to medium-low. Simmer for 2–3 minutes. Add the sea salt, cover, reduce the flame to low, and simmer for about 10 minutes, stirring occasionally. Place in serving bowls. Garnish with pieces of toasted nori and chopped parsley.

Creamy Buckwheat Soup

4–5 cups water or kombu soup stock (see page 104)
1/2 cup buckwheat groats, roasted
(see page 50 for roasting instructions)
1/8 teaspoon sea salt
1/2 cup onions, diced
1/4 cup celery, diced
Chopped parsley for garnish

Yield: 4–5 cup servings

Place the water or soup stock in a pot, cover, and bring to a boil. Add the buckwheat and a pinch or two of sea salt. Reduce the flame to medium-low, cover, and simmer for 10 minutes. Place the onions and celery in the pot and add the remaining sea salt. Cover and simmer for another 10 minutes. Place in serving bowls and garnish with chopped parsley.

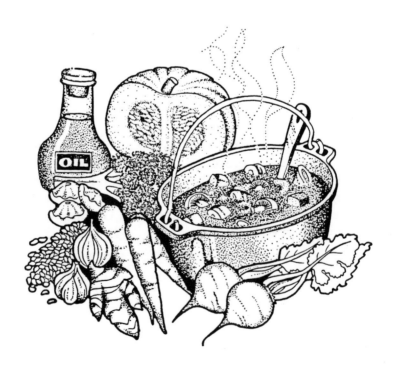

Chapter Six

FRESH MORNING VEGETABLES

Fresh vegetables are perfect as side dishes for breakfast. They are rich sources of complex carbohydrates, fiber, vitamins, and minerals. As part of a balanced diet, they help provide all of the nutrients that are essential for health and vitality. They go very well with porridge and soup in the morning. As you can see in the list of recommended vegetables in Chapter Two, there are many healthful varieties to choose from. Table 6.1 lists nutrients found in commonly used vegetables.

In recent times, however, the quality of vegetables and other farm and garden produce has declined considerably. This is largely due to modern agricultural practices, including the use of petroleum-based fertilizers, chemical pesticides, and other artificial sprays. Moreover, advances in refrigeration, canning, freezing, and transcontinental and intercontinental shipping have now virtually eliminated the traditional reliance on locally grown, fresh produce.

Meanwhile, with the spread of monocropping and other modern agricultural methods in the twentieth century, the demand has accelerated for uniform crops that can be grown, harvested, packaged, and shipped both quickly and inexpensively. With the practice of artificial hybridization of seeds, most traditional seed strains have disappeared and the food sold in supermarkets is largely the same in shape, size, color, and taste. Soil erosion, the evolution of insects resistant to pesticides, and other results of chemical farming have intensified the search for the perfect species of hybrid plants. Modern vegetables and other fruits of the earth are a pale reflection of their natural forebears.

Table 6.1   Nutrients in Commonly Used Vegetables

Nutrient	Good Sources
Complex carbohydrates	winter squash, broad beans, burdock, dandelion greens, ginger root, green peas, lotus root shiitake mushrooms, onions, parsley, parsnips
Fiber	broad beans, broccoli, Brussels sprouts, burdock, carrots, cauliflower, collard greens, daikon leaves, dandelion greens, ginger root, green peas, kale, lotus root, mustard greens, parsley, parsnips, pumpkin, scallions, winter squash
Vitamin A	broccoli, carrots, daikon, dandelion greens, kale, mustard greens, winter squash
Vitamin C	broccoli, Brussels sprouts, cabbage leaves, cauliflower, chives, collard greens
Calcium	broccoli, collard greens, daikon leaves, dried daikon, dandelion greens, watercress

Fortunately, the pendulum may now be swinging in the other direction as consumers become more aware of the potentially harmful effects of chemicalized food and start to demand organic produce. The importance of organic farming is also gaining official recognition. In 1989, the National Academy of Sciences issued a report recommending that American agriculture begin shifting toward natural and organic methods. Recent studies have also shown that organic farming is cost effective and competitive with nonorganic methods. It is also not ecologically destructive. Macrobiotic nutritional guidelines have long advocated the use of organic or natural-quality vegetables as much as possible, and suggest relying on locally grown produce in season. Canned and frozen vegetables are not recommended, nor are, for people in temperate zones, vegetables from tropical climates.

Tropical and semitropical vegetables may be enjoyed in their native setting, but are generally too extreme for use in four-season climates. This includes some species that originally came from southern latitudes, but are now grown in northern climates. In most cases, they have been cultivated in the new environment for only a few centuries, which, in evolutionary terms, is very brief. Among tropical vegetables, the solanaceous plants, also known as the nightshades, are especially unsuitable. These include many varieties used in modern temperate-climate breakfasts, such as potatoes, tomatoes, and green and red peppers, as well as cayenne pepper, eggplant, chili pepper, and paprika. Vegetables in the nightshade family are now being associated with a variety of illnesses, including arthritis. Dr. Norman Childers, a professor of horticulture at Cook College in New Jersey, has worked with solanaceous plants all of his life. He reported in his book *The Nightshades and Health* that many arthritic patients experienced the relief of symptoms once they eliminated the nightshades from their diets.

Plants of the goosefoot family are also generally avoided in macrobiotic kitchens. These vegetables of semitropical origin include spinach, Swiss chard, beets, lamb's quarters, and rhubarb. They are usually astringent to the taste, become dark when cooked, and do not combine well with other foods. In addition, they contain oxalic acid, which prevents the body from properly absorbing calcium into the cells and tissues. In extreme cases, oxalates can lead to the formation of calcium deposits in the joints or stones in the kidneys.

VEGETABLE CATEGORIES

Macrobiotic cooks often divide vegetables into three categories depending upon their direction of growth: leafy greens that branch upward above the soil, round-shaped or ground varieties that grow in or near the soil's surface, and root vegetables that grow deep within the earth. In terms of their energy qualities, leafy greens, such as kale and Chinese cabbage, are generally more yin or expansive; root vegetables, like carrots and turnips, are more yang or contractive; and round-shaped varieties, such as cabbage and squash, are in–between. Let us see how all three categories can be used in macrobiotic breakfasts.

Leafy greens. Greens such as kale; watercress; carrot, daikon, and turnip tops; and broccoli are used often in side dishes at breakfast. Their strong, upward energy goes well with the atmosphere in the morning, and they are quick and easy to make. Greens can be quickly boiled, steamed, or sautéed at breakfast. They complement the energy of soups and porridges, and add freshness to your meal. Chopped, fresh scallions are often used to garnish morning soups and porridges.

Round-Shaped or Ground Vegetables. Although they are delicious in side dishes, these vegetables are used more often in soups and porridges. Squash, cabbage, and onions, for example, are regular ingredients in morning miso soup. These vegetables often have naturally sweet flavors and add calming or centering energy to your meal.

Root Vegetables. Roots, such as carrots and daikon radish, are also used often in soups and porridges. They take longer to cook than leafy greens and are used more often in side dishes at other meals, although they can be quickly steamed or boiled to make delicious breakfast dishes. These vegetables have strong downward energy that activates and strengthens physical vitality. Generally, we do not recommend peeling root vegetables, unless you are using nonorganic or waxed varieties.

Cooking Whole or Slicing

As seen in Chapter Three, vegetables and other foods can be sliced in a variety of ways. Some vegetables, especially leafy greens, are also delicious when cooked whole and then sliced after cooking. Cooking leafy greens this way causes them to retain more of their nutrients and natural flavors. Thinly sliced vegetables are often better in dishes that require less time to prepare, since they cook more rapidly. Larger or thicker cuts are more appropriate in dishes that require a longer time to cook. In any case, don't stick with only one method of cutting or cooking your vegetables at breakfast. Each style or method imparts a slightly different taste, texture, and energy quality to the dish and, for optimal variety, we recommend using a range of cooking and cutting methods at each meal.

Using Leftovers

Leftovers from dinner can be recycled into breakfast or lunch on the following day. Leftover vegetables can simply be reheated or eaten, as is, at breakfast. Since cooked vegetables spoil after a certain time, especially in warm weather, it is best to store them overnight in the refrigerator or a cool pantry. Leftover greens can simply be removed from the refrigerator or pantry and allowed to sit for several minutes, until they reach room temperature. Root or ground vegetables may need to be quickly reheated before you eat them. They can be placed in a saucepan with a little water and heated for several minutes or quickly steamed before being served.

Breakfast Cooking Methods

The cooking methods used most often at breakfast include quick-boiling or blanching, quick-sautéing or stir-frying, pressing, steaming, and pickling. In the recipes that follow, guidelines are presented for using each of these methods in your morning meal.

Quick-Boiling (Blanching)

Quickly boiled or blanched vegetables add a light, fresh quality to morning meals. They are quick and simple to make, and are easy to digest. Blanched vegetables have a mild, often sweet, taste. Following are a variety of quickly boiled vegetable side dishes for use at breakfast.

Boiled Kale

Water
4–5 kale leaves
Small pinch of sea salt (optional)
Roasted sesame seeds for garnish (optional)
Umeboshi vinegar (optional)

Serves: 3–4

Place about 1/2 inch of water in a pot, cover, and bring to a boil. Wash the kale and remove the stem from the leaf. Slice the stem on a very thin diagonal. Slice the leafy portion into 1/2-inch strips or 1–inch squares. Keep the prepared leaves and stems separate. Place a small pinch of sea salt in the boiling water. Add the stems, cover, and boil 1–2 minutes. Remove with a spoon, place in a colander, and allow to cool. Place the sliced kale leaves in the same boiling water, cover, and cook for 1–2 minutes. Remove, place in a colander, and allow to cool. Place the stems and leaves in a serving bowl and mix together. Serve plain or with a few roasted sesame seeds sprinkled on top. A drop or two of umeboshi vinegar may also be added.

Ohatashi-Style Watercress

2 cups watercress
Water

Serves: 3–4

Place 1 inch of water in a pot, cover, and bring to a boil. Next add the washed watercress to the boiling water, cover, bring to a boil again, and cook for 40–45 seconds. Remove, place in a colander and allow to cool naturally or rinse quickly under cold water to stop the cooking action. Remove from the strainer, slice, and serve.

Boiled Carrots and Carrot Tops

Water
1/2 bunch carrots (sliced into thin rounds)
and their tops (finely sliced)
1/2 cup roasted sesame seeds (see page 50 for roasting instructions)
Tamari soy sauce

Serves: 3–4

Place 1 inch of water in a pot, cover, and bring to a boil. Place the carrots in the boiling water, cover, and simmer for 2–3 minutes until tender. Remove to a strainer, drain, and place in a bowl. Bring the water back to a boil and add the carrot tops. Cover and simmer for 1–1 1/2 minutes. Remove, place in a strainer, and drain. Mix together with the carrots. Place the roasted sesame seeds in a suribachi and partially grind. Add several drops of tamari soy sauce for a mild, salty flavor, and mix well. Mix the sesame seeds together with the carrots and carrot tops. Place in a serving bowl.

Instead of sesame seeds, try dry-roasting pumpkin seeds. Chop and grind them in a suribachi then mix them with the carrots and tops. You can use turnip and turnip greens in place of carrots. Boiled parsley prepared in this manner is also delicious.

Boiled Parsley with Pumpkin Seeds

1/2 cup roasted pumpkin seeds (see page 50 for roasting instructions)
Tamari soy sauce (optional)
Water
1 bunch fresh parsley

Serves: 3–4

Place the roasted pumpkin seeds on a cutting board and chop. Next, put them in a suribachi and grind several minutes. Add several drops of tamari soy sauce for a mild, salty flavor.

Place about 1 inch of water in a pot, cover, and bring to a boil. Place the washed, whole parsley in the boiling water, cover, and boil 1–2 minutes. Remove, drain, and allow to cool as is, or rinse quickly under cold water.

Place on a cutting board and finely slice or mince. Place the parsley in the suribachi with the roasted, ground pumpkin seeds, mix, and place in a serving bowl.

Mixed Boiled Vegetables

1/2 cup onions, sliced into thin half-moons
1/4 cup celery, cut into thin diagonals
1 cup gold nugget, red kuri, or buttercup squash, cut into
1/4-inch-thick wedges
1 cup carrots, cut into thin diagonals
Water
1/4 cup leeks, cut into 1/2-inch slices
Tamari soy sauce (optional)

Serves: 3–4

Layer the vegetables in a pot in the following manner: onions on the bottom, followed by the celery, the squash, and topped with the carrots. Add 1/2 inch of water, cover, and bring to a boil. Reduce the flame and simmer for 3–4 minutes. Place the leeks on top of the other vegetables, add 2–3 drops of tamari soy sauce, cover, and simmer for another 2–3 minutes. Remove the vegetables and place in a serving dish.

Boiled Salad

Water
1/2 cup yellow summer squash, sliced into 1/4-inch rounds or half rounds
1 cup cauliflower flowerets
1 cup broccoli flowerets
1/2 cup red radishes, halved

Serves: 3–4

Place 2–3 inches of water in a pot, cover, and bring to a boil. First, place the summer squash in the water, cover, and boil for 1–2 minutes, remove, and drain. Next, place the cauliflower in the same boiling water, cover, and boil for 2–3 minutes. Remove, drain, and place in the bowl together with the summer squash. Next, boil the broccoli flowerets for 2–3 minutes. Remove, place in a strainer, quickly rinse under cold water, and mix in with the other cooked vegetables. Finally, place the halved radishes in the boiling water, cover, and simmer for 1–2 minutes. Remove, place in a strainer, and drain. Mix the radishes together with the other vegetables and place in a serving bowl. Serve as is, or with condiments, roasted seeds, or your favorite dressing.

Boiled Watercress, Carrots, and Tofu Cubes

Water
1/2 cup fresh, firm-style tofu, cubed
1/2 cup carrots, sliced into thin half-moons
1 bunch watercress, cut into 1-inch lengths

Serves: 3–4

Place 1 inch of water in a pot, cover, and bring to a boil. Place the tofu in the boiling water, cover, and simmer 1 minute. Remove, drain in a strainer, and place in a bowl. Next, place the carrots in the boiling water, cover, and boil for 1–2 minutes until tender. Remove, drain in a strainer, and place in the bowl with the tofu. Place the watercress in the boiling water, cover, bring to a boil, and boil for 40–45 seconds. Remove, place in a strainer, and quickly rinse under cold water. Place the watercress in the bowl with the tofu and carrots. Mix and serve as is, or sprinkled with your favorite condiment.

Boiled Scallions or Leeks with Tempeh

Water
1/2 pound tempeh, cut into 1-inch cubes
2 slices fresh ginger
1 bunch of scallions or 1 stalk of leeks, cut into 1/2-inch lengths
Tamari soy sauce (optional)

Serves: 3–4

Place the tempeh in a saucepan with enough water to cover. Add the ginger slices. Cover the saucepan, bring to a boil, and reduce the flame to medium-low. Simmer the tempeh for about 20 minutes. Set the scallions or leeks on top of the tempeh. Add several drops of tamari soy sauce for a mild taste, cover, and let the scallions cook for 1–2 minutes. If using leeks, cook an additional 2–3 minutes until tender, but still bright green in color. Remove the ginger slices and discard. Place the tempeh and scallions, or leeks, in a serving dish.

Boiled Cabbage with Umeboshi

Water
1 umeboshi plum
2–3 cups green head cabbage, cut into 1-inch chunks

Serves: 3–4

Place the umeboshi plum and cabbage in a pot. Add about 1/2 inch of water, cover, and bring to a boil. Reduce the flame to medium-low and simmer for 4–5 minutes until the cabbage is tender. Remove and place in a serving bowl.

Boiled Daikon and Daikon Greens

1 strip kombu, 2 inches long, soaked and cut into
1/2-inch squares (see inset on page 87)
2 cups daikon (1 medium), cut into 1-inch-thick rounds
Water
Tamari soy sauce
1 cup daikon greens

Serves: 3–4

Place the kombu on the bottom of a saucepan with the daikon rounds on top. Add enough cold water to half-cover the daikon, cover the saucepan, and bring to a boil. Reduce the flame to medium-low and simmer for about 30 minutes. Add several drops of tamari soy sauce and set the daikon greens on top of the daikon rounds. Cover and simmer for another 3–4 minutes. Remove and place in a serving bowl.

For variety, try any of the following combinations: turnip and turnip greens, carrots and carrot tops, or rutabaga and rutabaga tops.

Quick-Sautéing or Stir-Frying

You can quick-sauté or stir-fry with high-quality sesame oil, or if you wish to limit your intake of oil, spring water can be used. Oil can be difficult to digest early in the morning, so we suggest using small amounts only, or eating a small serving of pickles or grated daikon to help balance the oil. Adding a drop or two of fresh ginger juice to the dish at the end of cooking also makes the oil more digestible. Vegetables may be seasoned with a small pinch of sea salt at the beginning of cooking, or with several drops of tamari soy sauce at the end. If you are sautéing with oil, it is best to season the dish lightly with either sea salt or tamari soy sauce, as these help create balance. Seasoning is not always necessary when you water sauté. Water-sautéed vegetables can simply be eaten as is.

Sautéed Chinese Cabbage

Dark sesame oil
3 cups Chinese cabbage leaves, halved and then sliced into
1/2-inch diagonals
Pinch of sea salt

Serves: 3–4

Brush a small amount of oil in a skillet and heat up over a high flame. Add the cabbage and a small pinch of sea salt. Move the vegetables around in the skillet with chopsticks or a wooden spoon for 1–2 minutes. Cover the skillet, reduce the flame to medium-low, and simmer for 2–3 minutes until tender, but still brightly colored. Remove and place in a serving dish.

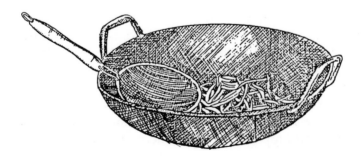

Stir-Fried Chinese Vegetables and Tofu

Dark sesame oil
1/4 cup fresh shiitake mushrooms, cut into 1/4-inch-thick slices
1/4 cup onions, sliced into thin half-moons
1/4 cup celery, sliced into thin diagonals
1/2 cup carrots, cut into matchsticks
1 cup bok choy, sliced into 1/2-inch diagonals
1/4 cup mung bean sprouts
1/2 cup fresh tofu, cubed
Tamari soy sauce
1/2 teaspoon fresh ginger juice

Serves: 3–4

Place all vegetables and tofu on a plate, keeping them separate from one another. Place a small amount of oil in a wok and place on a high flame. Heat the oil, but do not let it smoke. Add the shiitake and stir constantly for several seconds. Then add the onions and celery, stirring constantly for 1–2 minutes. Next, add the carrots and bok choy and stir for 2–3 minutes. Finally, add the mung bean sprouts, the tofu cubes, and several drops of tamari soy sauce. Cover the wok and let the sprouts and tofu steam for 1–2 minutes. Add the ginger juice, mix, and sauté several seconds more. Remove and place in a serving bowl.

Water-Sautéed Turnip or Daikon Greens

Water
3–4 cups turnip or daikon greens, sliced into 1-inch lengths
Tamari soy sauce (optional)

Serves: 3–4

Place enough water in a skillet to just cover the bottom, and bring to a boil. Add the greens and sauté for 1–2 minutes. Cover the skillet, reduce the flame to medium-low, and simmer for another 1–2 minutes. Add several drops of tamari soy sauce for a mild flavor, turn the flame up high, and cook off all remaining liquid, stirring the greens constantly. Remove and place in a serving bowl.

Sautéed Celery and Bean Sprouts

Dark sesame oil
1 cup celery, sliced into thin diagonals
2 cups mung bean sprouts
Water
Tamari soy sauce

Serves: 3–4

Heat a small amount of sesame oil in the bottom of a skillet. Add the celery and sauté 1–2 minutes. Next, add the bean sprouts, 2–3 drops of water, and several drops of tamari soy sauce for a mild flavor. Cover, reduce the flame to medium-low, and simmer for 2–3 minutes until the vegetables are tender, but still slightly crisp. Remove and place in a serving dish.

Water-Sautéed Mixed Vegetables

Water
1 cup onions, cut into 1/4-inch-thick wedges
1/2 cup carrots, sliced into thin matchsticks
1 cup cabbage, cut into 1-inch squares
1/2 cup leeks or scallions, cut into 1-inch lengths
Tamari soy sauce

Serves: 3–4

Place enough water in a skillet to just cover the bottom, and bring to a boil. Add the onions and sauté for 1–2 minutes, then add the carrots and cabbage. Sauté 1–2 minutes. Cover the skillet, reduce the flame to medium-low, and simmer 3–4 minutes. Add the leeks or scallions and sprinkle several drops of tamari soy sauce on top of the vegetables. Cover and simmer another 1–2 minutes. Remove the cover, mix the vegetables together, turn up the flame, and cook off any remaining liquid. Remove and place in a serving dish.

Sautéed Parsnips and Carrots

Dark sesame oil
1 1/2 cups parsnips, shaved
1 1/2 cups carrots, sliced into thin matchsticks
Pinch of sea salt
Water
Chopped parsley for garnish

Serves: 3–4

Heat a small amount of oil in a skillet. Add the parsnips and sauté 1–2 minutes. Layer the carrots on top of the parsnips, without mixing. Add a pinch of sea salt and several drops of water, and cover. Reduce the flame to medium-low and simmer for several minutes until tender and sweet. Remove the cover, turn up the flame, mix the vegetables together, and cook off any remaining liquid. Place in a serving dish and garnish with a small amount of chopped parsley.

Steaming

Steamed vegetables can add a light, refreshing quality to breakfasts. They are also quick and easy to make. Bitter vegetables such as dandelions, daikon greens, watercress, escarole, endive, chicory, turnip greens, carrot tops, and parsley are better when boiled. Steaming may cause them to become more bitter, while boiling tends to remove some of the bitter taste. Milder- or sweeter-tasting vegetables become sweeter when steamed. Vegetables can be steamed in several ways:

With a Collapsible Steamer Basket. Place the steamer at the bottom of a pot with about 1/2 inch of water. Cover the pot and bring the water to a boil. Add the vegetables and steam from several seconds to several minutes, depending on their size, thickness, or toughness.

With a Bamboo Steamer. Set the bamboo steamer on top of a pot with about a 1/2 inch of water and bring the water to a boil. Place the vegetables in the basket, put the cover on top, and steam as above.

In a Pot or Skillet. Place enough cold water in a skillet or pot to barely cover the bottom. Bring to a boil, place the vegetables inside, cover the skillet or pot, and quickly steam over a high flame until the vegetables are tender.

Steamed Chinese Cabbage with Mochi

4 leaves of Chinese cabbage, whole
4 pieces of mochi, 2 × 3 × 1/2 inch (see recipe on page 67)
Water

Yield: 4 stuffed cabbage leaves

Place enough water in a skillet to cover the bottom. Cover and bring to a boil. Place 1 piece of mochi on top of each cabbage leaf (near the bottom portion of the leaf). Fold the leaf over and cover the mochi, creating a sandwich effect. Place the mochi-stuffed leaves in the skillet, cover, and steam for 2–3 minutes until the leaves are tender and the mochi has melted inside the leaves. Remove the stuffed leaves and eat whole, or slice each stuffed leaf into quarters.

Regular green cabbage leaves may be used instead of Chinese cabbage, but they require a little longer cooking time as their leaves are tougher. You can also place diced vegetables or sweet corn on top of the mochi before steaming. They will cook into the mochi as the leaves steam.

Steamed Winter Squash

Water
2–3 cups buttercup, butternut, Hokkaido pumpkin, gold nugget, red kuri,
or other winter squash, cut into 1-inch chunks
Small pinch of sea salt or a couple drops of tamari soy sauce (optional)

Serves: 3–4

Place 1/2 inch of water in a pot. Set a stainless steel, collapsible steamer basket inside the pot. Cover the pot and bring the water to a boil. Place the squash inside the steamer basket. Sprinkle a pinch of sea salt or a few drops of tamari soy sauce on top, if desired. Cover and steam several minutes until the squash is soft. Remove and place in a serving dish.

Steamed Kale and Carrots

Water
1 cup carrots, cut into thin diagonals
2 cups kale, sliced into 1-inch pieces

Serves: 3–4

Place 1/2–1 inch of water in a pot. Set a bamboo steamer on top of the pot. Cover the steamer and bring the water to a boil. Place the carrots in the steamer, cover, and steam 2–3 minutes until tender. Remove and place in a bowl. Next, place the kale in the steamer. Cover and steam for 1–2 minutes until tender, but still bright green in color. Remove and mix in with the carrots. Serve hot.

Steamed Sweet Corn

Water
2 ears fresh sweet corn, husked and broken in half
3 umeboshi plums

Serves: 2

At the bottom of a pot, place a stainless steel steamer basket along with 1/2 inch of water. Cover and bring the water to a boil. Place the sweet corn in the basket, cover, and steam 3–5 minutes until tender and sweet. Remove and place on a serving platter. When served, rub a little umeboshi plum on each piece of sweet corn before eating.

Steamed Cabbage and Sauerkraut

Water
2 1/2 cups green head cabbage, cut into 1-inch pieces
1/2 cup sauerkraut

Serves: 3–4

Place 1/2 inch of water in a pot, set a steamer basket inside, cover, and bring the water to a boil. Place the cabbage in the steamer and set the sauerkraut on top of the cabbage. Cover the pot and steam 4–5 minutes until the cabbage is tender, but still bright green. Remove and place in a serving bowl.

Pressing

Depending on the texture of the vegetables you use and how you slice them, pressed vegetables can be ready in anywhere from 1–3 hours. They can also be left for 2–3 days, in which case they become more like pickles. Most pressed vegetables are very thinly sliced to reduce pressing time. They can be made ahead of time and simply served at breakfast.

Fresh produce is very important in producing the most flavorful pressed dishes. Older, drier vegetables have a lower water content and may be tougher, detracting from the taste of the dish and lengthening the amount of time needed for them to be ready. Vegetables are usually pressed with flavor enhancers such as sea salt, tamari soy sauce, brown rice or sweet brown rice vinegar, mirin (sweet rice cooking wine), umeboshi plums, or umeboshi vinegar. These initiate fermentation, making the vegetables more digestible. If your pressed vegetables taste overly salty, simply place them in a strainer and rinse quickly under cold water. Pressed vegetables can also be eaten at lunch or dinner. About 1/3 cup per day is usually sufficient.

Pressed vegetables can be made in two basic ways. The first is with a pickle press. This is a special plastic jar with a lid that screws on and a pressure plate for applying pressure. After washing and cutting your vegetables, place them in the press with one of the seasonings described above. Fasten the lid and tighten the pressure plate. Simply let them sit for the amount of time indicated in the recipe. Pickle presses are available in most natural foods stores. If you don't have a pickle press, simply place the sliced vegetables and seasoning in a bowl and put a plate on top. Place some type of weight on top of the plate to apply pressure, and let your vegetables sit for the amount of time indicated in the recipe.

Pressed Carrot and Daikon

1 cup carrots, sliced into very thin matchsticks
1 cup daikon, sliced into very thin matchsticks
1/4 teaspoon sea salt
2 tablespoons brown rice vinegar

Serves: 3–4

Thoroughly mix the vegetables, sea salt, and vinegar in a pickle press. Allow the vegetables to press for 1–2 hours. Remove and squeeze out any excess liquid. If too salty for your taste, rinse quickly under cold water. Place in a serving dish.

Mixed Vegetable Pressed Salad

2 cups Chinese cabbage, sliced into very thin diagonals
1/4 cup red radishes, sliced into very thin rounds
1/4 cup red onion, sliced into thin half-moons or half-rings
1/4 cup celery, cut into thin diagonals
1/4 cup red radish tops, cut into 1/2-inch lengths
1 tablespoon sweet brown rice vinegar
1/4–1/2 teaspoon sea salt

Serves: 3–4

Place all ingredients in a pickle press, mix together thoroughly, and apply pressure for 1–2 hours. Remove and squeeze out any excess liquid. If too salty, rinse quickly under cold water. Place in a serving dish.

Lettuce Pressed Salad

2 cups lettuce (any type), finely shredded
1/2 cucumber, sliced into thin half-moons
1/4 cup carrots, coarsely grated
1 tablespoon chopped parsley, minced
1 tablespoon roasted black sesame seeds (see page 50 for roasting
instructions)
2 tablespoons umeboshi vinegar

Serves: 3–4

Place the vegetables, roasted sesame seeds, and umeboshi vinegar in a pickle press. Mix thoroughly, cover, and apply pressure. Let sit for 1 hour. Remove, squeeze out excess water, and if too salty, rinse quickly under cold water. Place in a serving dish.

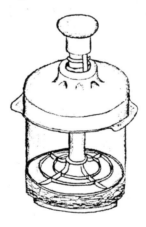

Simple Salt-Pressed Cabbage

3 cups cabbage, finely shredded
1/4–1/2 teaspoon sea salt

Serves: 3–4

Place the cabbage and sea salt in a pickle press and mix thoroughly. Cover the press, apply pressure, and let sit for about 3 hours. Remove and squeeze out any excess liquid. Rinse quickly under cold water if too salty. Place in a serving dish.

Pressed Daikon in Lemon Juice

2 cups daikon, sliced into thin rounds or half-rounds
1 teaspoon fresh lemon juice
1/4 teaspoon sea salt
1 tablespoon roasted black sesame seeds (see page 50 for roasting
instructions)

Serves: 3–4

Place the daikon, lemon juice, and sea salt in a pickle press and mix thoroughly. Cover the press, apply pressure, and let sit for 2–3 hours. Remove from the press and squeeze out any excess liquid. Rinse if too salty. Place in a serving bowl and garnish with the roasted black sesame seeds.

Marinated Lotus Root and Parsley

This recipe does not require pressing,however, the slight fermentation caused by the marinating mixture is similar to that which occurs when pressing vegetables.

1 cup fresh lotus root, quartered and sliced as thinly as possible
1 1/2 teaspoons tamari soy sauce
1 tablespoon brown rice vinegar
1 tablespoon mirin
1 teaspoon minced parsley

Yield: Approximately 1 cup

Place all of the ingredients together in a bowl. Let sit for 1 hour, mixing once or twice. Drain and place in a serving dish.

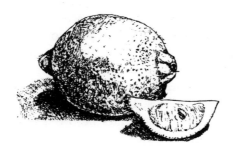

Pressed Red Radishes

1 medium-sized bunch or a 6-ounce package of red radishes,
sliced into very thin rounds
1 bunch red radish tops (optional), cut into 1/4-inch lengths
2 tablespoons umeboshi vinegar

Yield: Approximately 2 cups

Place all ingredients in a pickle press, mix thoroughly, and cover. Apply pressure and allow to sit for 2–3 hours. Remove, rinse if too salty, squeeze out excess liquid, and place in a serving dish.

Tamari Pressed Onions

Water
2 cups onions, sliced into very thin half-moons
1 1/2 tablespoons tamari soy sauce

Yield: Approximately 1 1/2–2 cups

Place 1/2 inch of water in a saucepan, cover, and bring to a boil. Place the onions in, cover, and blanch for 30 seconds. Remove, place in a strainer, and rinse quickly under cold water. Place the onions and tamari soy sauce in a pickle press, mix thoroughly, and cover the press. Screw down cover to apply pressure and let sit for 2–3 hours. Remove, rinse if too salty, squeeze out excess liquid, and place in a serving bowl.

Pickling

Pickled vegetables are similar to those that are pressed. The main differences are that pickling takes longer and uses a larger quantity of salt. Whole, unsliced vegetables are also used, occasionally, in making pickles. As with pressed vegetables, pickles are usually made in advance and then served at breakfast. About 1 tablespoonful or so is usually enough per serving. In the following recipes we show how to make quick-, medium-, and long-term pickles. If your pickles have an overly salty taste, simply rinse them under cold water before serving.

Quick Tamari-Rutabaga Pickles

2 cups rutabaga, cut into very thin slices
1–1 1/2 cups water
1/3–1/2 cup tamari soy sauce

Yield: Approximately 2–3 cups

Place all ingredients in a clean glass jar, cover, and shake to thoroughly mix. Let sit for as little as 3–4 hours, or as long as 3–4 days. The longer they sit, the saltier the pickles will become. Remove, place in a strainer, rinse quickly under cold water, and place in a serving dish.

Try very thinly sliced carrots, onions, daikon, or turnips, instead of rutabaga, using the same proportions as above. For a sweeter-tasting onion pickle, quickly blanch the onions and rinse under cold water before pickling.

Quick Red Radish-Umeboshi Pickles

5–6 umeboshi plums
2 quarts water
1–2 cups whole, red radishes

Yield: Approximately 1–2 cups

Place the umeboshi and water in a saucepan, cover, and bring to a boil. Reduce the flame and simmer for 4–5 minutes. Remove from the flame and allow to cool completely. Place the radishes in a clean glass jar. Pour the cooled umeboshi liquid and plums into the glass jar, covering the radishes. Place a lid on the radishes, shake to mix, and let sit for 3–5 days. Refrigerate when done pickling. Before serving, remove, rinse, and slice. The pickles will keep, refrigerated, for about 3–4 weeks. The longer they sit, the saltier and more sour they will become.

Quick Salt-Brine Pickles

5–6 cups water
1/8–1/4 cup sea salt
2 pickling cucumbers, quartered or cut into 1/4-inch-thick rounds
1/2 cup onions, cut into 1/4-inch wedges or half-moons
1/2 cup broccoli flowerets
1/2 cup cauliflower flowerets
1/4 cup carrots, cut into thin diagonals
1–2 sprigs fresh dill (optional)
1/8 cup sauerkraut

Yield: 4 cups

Place all of the ingredients in a large, clean glass jar. Mix thoroughly. Cover the mouth of the jar with a piece of cotton cheesecloth to keep dust out. Set aside for 2–4 days in a cool, dry place. Cover the jar with a lid and refrigerate for 1–3 days. The pickles are now ready to rinse under cold water and serve. They will keep in the refrigerator for approximately 1 month.

Turnip-Kombu Salt Pickles

1 strip kombu (4 inches long), soaked and sliced into very thin matchsticks
2–3 cups white or purple-top turnips, sliced into paper-thin
rounds or half-moons
1/2 teaspoon sea salt

Yield: Approximately 2–2 1/2 cups

Place the kombu and turnips in a pickle press. Add the sea salt and mix thoroughly. Cover, apply pressure, and let sit for 2–3 days. Remove, rinse, and place in a serving dish. These pickles will keep for several days in the refrigerator. If refrigerating for several days, it is best to remove them from the pickle press and place them in a tightly sealed glass jar.

Sweet and Sour Quick-Ginger Pickles

2 pieces fresh ginger (2–3 inches long), thinly sliced
1 tablespoon sweet brown rice vinegar
1 tablespoon mirin
2 tablespoons shiso leaves

Yield: Approximately 1 cup

Place the ginger in a pickle press. Add the mirin and vinegar. Mix well. Mix in the shiso leaves, cover, and apply pressure. Let sit for about 3–4 days or until the ginger turns pink and is slightly sweet, but sour. Remove, rinse, and serve.

Long-Term Nuka Pickles

2–3 heads Chinese cabbage
Sea salt
Organic nuka

Yield: 10–12 cups

Wash the cabbage and remove the leaves. Place the cabbage leaves in a dish drainer and set in the sun for 2 days to dry. Sprinkle a small amount of sea salt on the bottom of a pickle press. Layer the cabbage in the press, alternating the direction of the layers. Between each layer of leaves, sprinkle a small handful of sea salt. Repeat until all of the cabbage is used up. Sprinkle a small handful of sea salt on top of the last layer of cabbage. Cover and apply pressure. Set in a cool place for about 10 hours. The sea salt will draw out water from the cabbage. If the water level is not up to or above the lid within 10 hours, there is either not enough pressure or not enough sea salt. Apply more pressure or add more sea salt.

After 10 hours, if the water level has risen to the lid, pour off the salty water and discard. Remove the cabbage from the press. Place the nuka in a hot skillet and dry-roast for several minutes, until it releases a nutty fragrance (see page 50 for roasting instructions). Remember to stir constantly to prevent the nuka from burning. Sprinkle a layer of nuka on the bottom of the crock or keg. Next, layer the cabbage, in alternate directions again, but this time sprinkle a small handful of nuka between each layer of cabbage. Sprinkle nuka on top of the last layer of cabbage leaves. Cover and press again. Let sit for 7 days in a cool place. When ready, remove, rinse under cold water, slice, and eat.

Chinese cabbage salt pickles can be prepared in the same manner as above, omitting the use of nuka. Simply layer the cabbage and sea salt in a press, cover and apply pressure for 7 days. Remove, rinse, slice, and eat.

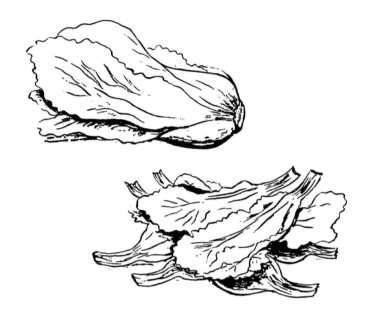

Chapter Seven

TOFU, SOY, AND WHOLE WHEAT PRODUCTS

For centuries, processed soybean and whole wheat products were an important part of traditional diets. Soyfoods like tofu and tempeh are very high in protein, contain no cholesterol, and are very low in saturated fat. They are delicious and can be made to taste like many familiar breakfast foods. Tofu, for example, is a very adaptable food and can be scrambled like eggs. Tofu can also be used to make creamy "cheese" or mouthwatering French toast. Seitan (naturally processed whole wheat gluten) and tempeh (fermented whole soybeans) have a taste and texture similar to meat. They can be delicious, healthy substitutes for high-cholesterol breakfast foods such as bacon, ham, and sausage. These traditional staple foods are now gaining popularity throughout the world as people search for low-fat, cholesterol-free alternatives in their diets.

Twenty years ago, when the natural food movement was just starting in this country, many of these foods had to be made at home. Now, more than 10,000 natural foods stores and cooperatives, throughout North America and Europe, carry these and other traditional, naturally processed foods. Today you can find ready-made tofu, tempeh, and seitan in the refrigerator cases of most natural foods stores as well as many supermarkets.

However, when buying tofu you need to be careful about quality. In a process similar to the curding of dairy cheese with rennet, traditionally made tofu is solidified from soy milk with a mineral-rich substance called *nigari*. Nigari is the concentrated residue remaining from sea salt that has been extracted from sea water; it is rich in magnesium and other mineral compounds. Another good-quality natural solidifier is unrefined calcium sulfate, which comes from the mineral gypsum. Today, most of the tofu sold in Oriental food stores is made with vinegar, alum, refined calcium sulfate, or other low-quality ingredients. Good-quality tofu should be made with organic soybeans and real nigari or natural calcium sulfate. If these are unavailable, lemon juice is the next best substitute for solidifying tofu.

Similarly, when you buy foods such as muffins, bread, bagels, and crackers to make special breakfast dishes, be sure to buy them at the natural foods store. These items should be made from unprocessed whole wheat flour and should be free of additives, honey, or refined sugar. Commercially baked goods are not ideal for maintaining optimal health. At the same time, dill pickles, sauerkraut, or seasonings such as miso mustard, should be natural and unprocessed. They can also be bought at natural foods stores. In some cases, especially when someone is starting macrobiotics for health reasons, it may be best to wait before using specialty foods such as these. If you are unsure about making the specialty dishes in this or other chapters in this book, check first with a macrobiotics teacher or counselor.

PREPARING TOFU AND TEMPEH

Preprocessed tofu, tempeh, and seitan don't need to be washed. Tempeh can be used as is from the package. When you buy tofu or seitan in containers, simply pour off the water before slicing. Dried tofu needs to be soaked before being added to recipes. Simply place the dried tofu in a bowl and add warm water to cover. Let it soak for 7–10 minutes. Pour off the soaking water. Then add cold water to cover, quickly rinse, and pour

Figure 7.1 Cutting Tofu

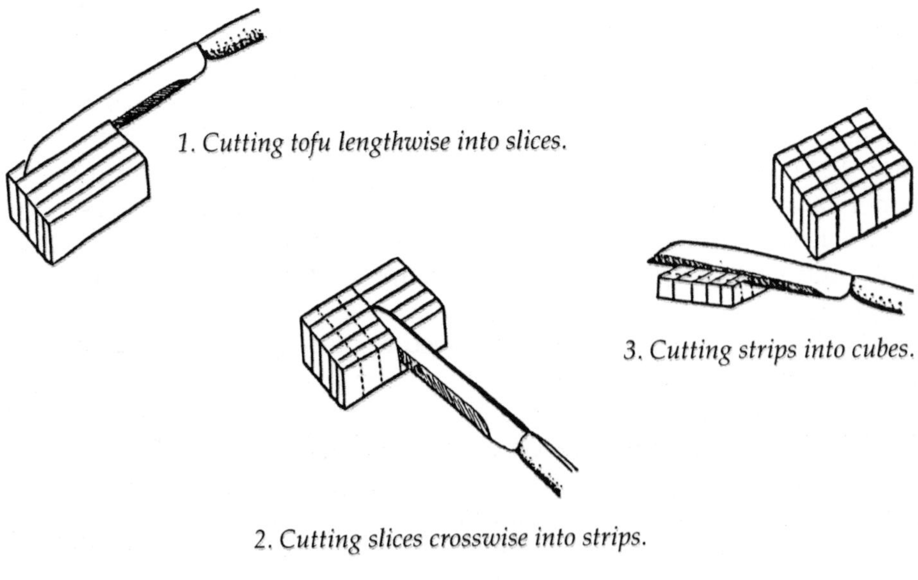

1. Cutting tofu lengthwise into slices.

3. Cutting strips into cubes.

2. Cutting slices crosswise into strips.

off. Stack two or three pieces on top of each other, squeeze out the excess liquid, and place on your cutting board.

As shown in Figure 7.1, to cut tofu into rectangular slices, place it on a cutting board and cut it crosswise into 1/4–1/2-inch slices. If you wish to make cubes, first cut the tofu crosswise, then cut it lengthwise into 1/2–1-inch strips. Then cut 2 or 3 strips at a time into 1-inch cubes. To cut dried tofu or tempeh, place on the cutting board and slice lengthwise into 1/4–1-inch strips. Then cut the strips, 2 or 3 at a time, into 1-inch cubes. Seitan can simply be sliced on the diagonal or cubed.

Plain Boiled Tofu

Water
1 cake fresh, firm-style tofu, (16 ounces), cubed
Tamari soy sauce (optional)
Chopped scallions for garnish

Serves: 4

Place 1/2 inch of water in a saucepan. Cover and bring to a boil. Place the tofu in the boiling water. Cover, reduce the flame to medium-low, and simmer for 1–2 minutes. Season with several drops of tamari soy sauce, cover, and simmer another minute. Remove, place in a serving dish, and garnish with chopped scallions.

Broiled Tofu Slices

1 cake fresh, firm-style tofu (16 ounces), cut into
1/4–1/2-inch-thick slices
Tamari soy sauce

Serves: 4

Place the tofu slices on an unoiled cookie sheet and sprinkle several drops of tamari soy sauce on each slice. Place the cookie sheet under the broiler and cook the tofu until slightly browned (3–5 minutes). Using a spatula, turn the slices over and brown the other side (2–3 minutes). Remove and place on a serving platter or use in making sandwiches.

Pan-Fried Tofu Slices

Light or dark sesame oil
1 cake fresh, firm-style tofu (16 ounces), cut into
1/4–1/2-inch-thick slices
Tamari soy sauce

Serves: 4

Brush a small amount of sesame oil in a skillet or on a pancake griddle and heat up. Place the tofu slices in and sprinkle 1–2 drops of tamari soy sauce on each slice. Pan-fry for 1–2 minutes. Turn the tofu over and sprinkle another 1–2 drops of the soy sauce on each slice. Fry 1–2 minutes. Turn the tofu over once again and fry another 1–2 minutes. Eat as is or use in making sandwiches.

Pan-Fried Tofu and Vegetables

Dark sesame oil
1/4 cup onion, diced
1/4 cup mushrooms, thinly sliced
1/4 cup green pepper, diced
1/4 cup carrots, cut into thin matchsticks
1/2 cake fresh, firm-style tofu (8 ounces), cubed
Tamari soy sauce

Serves: 4

Brush a small amount of oil in a skillet and heat up. Add the onions and sauté for 1 minute. Next, add the mushrooms and green pepper and sauté 1–2 minutes. Now, add the carrots and tofu to the skillet, along with several drops of tamari soy sauce. Cover and reduce the flame to medium-low. Simmer for 3–4 minutes until the tofu is soft and fluffy and the vegetables are tender. Gently mix the tofu and vegetables together and simmer, uncovered, another minute or so until all of the liquid has evaporated. Place in a serving dish.

For a variation, when in season, try adding fresh sweet corn, green beans, or scallions for a sweet and light tofu dish.

Scrambled Tofu and Celery

Dark sesame oil
1/2–1 cup celery, sliced into thin diagonals
1 cake fresh, firm-style tofu (16 ounces)
Sea salt
1 tablespoon sesame seeds, lightly roasted
(see page 50 for roasting instructions)

Serves: 4

Brush a small amount of sesame oil in a skillet, add the celery, and sauté for 1–2 minutes. Next, with your hands, squeeze and crumble the tofu over the celery. Add a pinch of sea salt, cover, and reduce the flame to medium-low. Simmer for 2–3 minutes or until the celery is tender and the tofu is light and fluffy. Remove the cover and cook off any remaining liquid. Place in a serving bowl and sprinkle the roasted sesame seeds on top.

Scrambled Tofu and Vegetables with Umeboshi Vinegar

Dark sesame oil
1/2 cup onion, diced
1 cup fresh sweet corn, removed from the cob
1 cake fresh, firm-style tofu (16 ounces)
2 tablespoons umeboshi vinegar
1/4 cup scallions, sliced

Serves: 4

Brush a small amount of oil on the bottom of a skillet. Add the onions and sauté 1–2 minutes. Layer the sweet corn on top of the onions. Next, with your hands, crumble the tofu on top of the sweet corn. Sprinkle the umeboshi vinegar on top of the tofu. Cover and reduce the flame to medium-low. Simmer for 3–5 minutes until the vegetables are tender and the tofu is light and fluffy. Add the scallions, cover, and cook for another 1–2 minutes. Remove and place in a serving dish.

Scrambled Tofu with Tamari Soy Sauce
and Vegetables

Dark sesame oil
1/4 cup onion, diced
1/4 cup carrots, cut into matchsticks
2 tablespoons burdock, shaved
1 cake fresh, firm-style tofu (16 ounces)
Tamari soy sauce
1/4 cup leeks, sliced into thin diagonals
1/4 cup almonds, slivered

Serves: 4

Brush a small amount of sesame oil in a skillet and heat up. Add the onions and sauté for 1 minute. Next, add the carrots and burdock and sauté for 1–2 minutes. Finally, crumble the tofu on top of the vegetables. Cover the skillet, reduce the flame to medium-low, and simmer 4–5 minutes until the vegetables are tender and the tofu is light and fluffy. Sprinkle several drops of tamari soy sauce on top of the tofu. Add the leeks and slivered almonds. Cover and simmer for another 1–2 minutes. Remove the cover, turn the flame to high, and cook off most of the remaining liquid. Place in a serving dish.

Oilless Scrambled Tofu and Vegetables

Water
1/4 cup onions, diced
1/2 cup fresh sweet corn, removed from the cob
1 cake fresh, firm-style tofu (16 ounces)
1/2 cup snow peas, de-stemmed and diagonally sliced in half
Tamari soy sauce

Serves: 4

Place a small amount of water in the bottom of a skillet, so that it just barely covers the bottom, and bring to a boil. Add the onions and sauté for 2–3 minutes (as you would if using oil), moving the onions around in the skillet. Layer the sweet corn on top of the onions and crumble the tofu on top of the vegetables, but do not mix together. Cover, bring to a boil, reduce the flame to medium-low, and simmer several minutes until the vegetables are tender and the tofu is light and fluffy. Remove the cover, add the snow peas, and sprinkle several drops of tamari soy sauce over the tofu. Cover and simmer another 2–3 minutes until the peas are tender, but still bright green. Remove the cover, turn the flame up, and cook off most of the remaining liquid. Mix the ingredients together and place in a serving bowl.

Tofu–Vegetable Roll

1 cake fresh, firm-style tofu (16 ounces)
1/4 cup fresh sweet corn, removed from the cob
4–5 fresh green beans, de-stemmed and thinly sliced on the diagonal
Tamari soy sauce

Yield: 8 slices

Place the tofu in a suribachi and grind to a thick purée. Next, add the corn, green beans, and several drops of tamari soy sauce to the suribachi. Mix. Take a bamboo sushi mat and lay it flat on your cutting surface. Put the puréed tofu mixture directly onto the mat so that only an inch at the top and 2 inches at the bottom are left uncovered. Roll the purée up inside the mat making sure the mat surrounds the cream, but does not get caught inside it. Figure 7.2 (page 142) illustrates this procedure. Place an inch of water in a pot and place a bamboo steamer on top. Bring to a boil and place the sushi mat, with the tofu inside it, in the steamer. Cover and steam for about 10–15 minutes. Remove the mat and unwind it, releasing the tofu inside. Place the tofu roll on a cutting board and slice in half. Slice each half again in half, then slice each quarter in half. You should now have eight pieces of tofu roll. Place on a serving platter, garnish, and serve.

Figure 7.2   Making a Tofu-Vegetable Roll

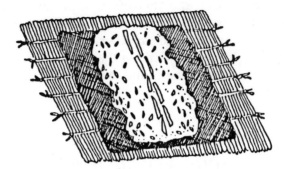

1. Tofu-vegetable mixture on a sushi mat.

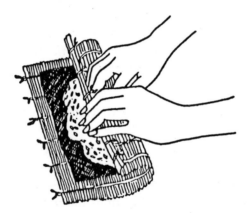

2. Rolling the tofu-vegetable mixture.

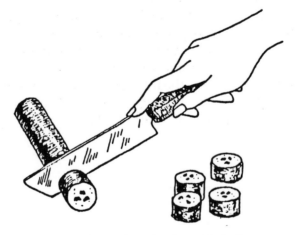

3. Slicing the Tofu-Vegetable Roll.

Sautéed Dried Tofu and Vegetables

1/2 package, dried tofu slices (2 1/2 ounces)
Dark sesame oil
1/4 cup onions, sliced into half-moons
1/2 cup Brussels sprouts, de-stemmed and cut in half
1/4 cup carrots, sliced into matchsticks
Water
Tamari soy sauce

Serves: 3–4

Soak the dried tofu according to the instructions found in Table 5.1 (page 89). Make sure all soaking and rinsing waters are discarded. After squeezing out any excess water, slice the soaked tofu into 1/4-inch-thick strips. Brush a small amount of oil in a skillet and heat up. Add the onion slices to the skillet and sauté for 1–2 minutes, then add the Brussels sprouts and carrots. Sauté 1 minute. Place the tofu slices on top of the vegetables. Add enough cold water to just cover the bottom of the skillet. Bring to a boil, cover, and reduce the flame to medium-low. Simmer for about 5–7 minutes until the vegetables and tofu are tender. Add several drops of tamari soy sauce, cover, and simmer another minute. Remove the cover, turn up the flame, and cook off any remaining liquid. Just before most of the liquid is gone, mix all of the ingredients together. Place in a serving bowl.

Boiled Dried Tofu and Scallions

Water
1/2 package dried tofu slices (2 1/2 ounces)
3 medium-sized scallions, chopped
Tamari soy sauce

Serves: 3–4

Soak the dried tofu slices according to the instructions found in Table 5.1 (page 89). Make sure all soaking and rinsing waters are discarded. Place the tofu in a saucepan and add enough cold water to half-cover the slices. Bring to a boil, cover, and reduce the flame to medium-low. Simmer for about 10–15 minutes. Add the scallions and several drops of tamari soy sauce to the saucepan. Cover and let simmer for 1–2 minutes. Remove the cover, turn the flame to high, and cook off any remaining liquid. Mix the scallions and tofu together and place in a serving bowl.

Tempeh and Onions

2 cups onions, sliced into 1/2-inch wedges
1 package tempeh (8 ounces), cut into 1-inch cubes
Water
Tamari soy sauce
Chopped parsley for garnish

Serves: 3–4

Place the onions on the bottom of a saucepan. Set the tempeh on top of the onions. Add water to half-cover the tempeh, cover, and bring to a boil. Reduce the flame to medium-low and simmer for 20–25 minutes. Add several drops of tamari soy sauce, cover, and simmer for another 5 minutes. Remove the cover, turn up the flame, and simmer until almost all remaining liquid is gone. Mix and place in a serving dish. Garnish with chopped parsley.

Pan-Fried Tempeh

Dark sesame oil
1 package tempeh (8 ounces), cut into 3 × 2 × 1/4-inch slices
Water
Tamari soy sauce

Serves: 3–4

Heat a small amount of sesame oil in a skillet. Add the tempeh slices and brown on each side. Add enough water to just cover. Bring to a boil in covered skillet. Reduce the flame to medium-low and simmer for about 20–25 minutes. Season with a few drops of tamari soy sauce and simmer another 5 minutes. Remove the cover, turn the flame to high, and cook off any remaining liquid. Pan-fried tempeh is great for making sandwiches; it can also be sliced into strips and served as is.

Tempeh and Sauerkraut

1 package tempeh (8 ounces), sliced into 1-inch cubes
1 cup green cabbage, shredded
1/2 cup sauerkraut
Water

Serves: 3–4

Place the tempeh on the bottom of a saucepan, layer the shredded cabbage on top, and cover the cabbage with the sauerkraut. Add enough water to half-cover the tempeh. Cover the pot and bring to a boil. Reduce the flame to medium-low and simmer for about 20 minutes. Remove the cover and cook off most of the remaining liquid. Place in a serving bowl.

Tempeh Sandwich

3–4 slices Pan-Fried Tempeh (see page 144), 3 × 2 × 1/4 inches
3–4 whole wheat bagels
3–4 cucumber slices
Lettuce leaves
Sauerkraut
Miso mustard (optional)

Yield: 3–4 bagel sandwiches

Slice the bagels in half and place the slices of pan-fried tempeh on the bottom halves. Garnish with a slice of cucumber, a small amount of sauerkraut, some lettuce, and a little miso mustard. Top with the remaining bagel halves and serve.

Pan-Fried Seitan Slices

Dark sesame oil
6–8 pieces fresh seitan, 1/4-inch-thick slices (see page 77 for recipe)
Parsley sprig for garnish

Serves: 3–4

Heat a small amount of oil in a skillet. Add the seitan slices and pan-fry on both sides until slightly browned. Remove, place on a platter, and garnish with a sprig of parsley. Pan-fried seitan slices also make great sandwiches.

Seitan and Sauerkraut

1 medium onion, sliced into 1/4-inch-thick rounds
6–8 pieces fresh seitan, 1/4-inch-thick slices (see page 77 for recipe)
1/2 cup sauerkraut
Water

Serves: 3–4

Place the onion rounds on the bottom of a skillet. Place the seitan slices on top of the onions and the sauerkraut on top of the seitan. Add enough water to just cover the onions. Cover the skillet, bring to a boil, and reduce the flame to medium-low. Simmer for about 7–10 minutes until the onions are soft and tender and the seitan is hot. Remove the cover, turn the flame up to high, and cook off the remaining liquid. At the last minute, just before all of the liquid is gone, mix the ingredients together and place in a serving bowl.

Tempeh, Mushrooms, and Celery

1 cup white mushrooms, de-stemmed and thinly sliced
1 cup celery, sliced into thin diagonals
1 package tempeh, (8 ounces), cut into 1-inch cubes
1 1/2 cups water
Tamari soy sauce
2 teaspoons kuzu

Serves: 3–4

Place the mushrooms, celery, and tempeh in a saucepan. Add the water, cover, and bring to a boil. Reduce the flame to medium low and simmer for about 20 minutes. Add a few drops of tamari soy sauce for a mild flavor and reduce the flame to low. Dilute the kuzu with a little water and add to the saucepan, stirring constantly to prevent lumping. When the kuzu becomes thick and translucent, remove and place in a serving dish.

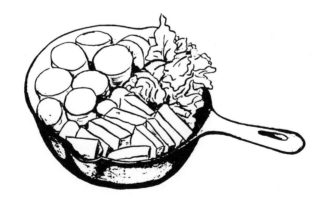

Chapter Eight
CONDIMENTS AND NATURAL SWEETENERS

Condiments and garnishes can be added to your breakfast dishes offering a good example of complementary balance. Most of the condiments used in macrobiotic cooking add taste, nutrients, and especially minerals to dishes. Although they contain a balance of energies, condiments are generally more contractive. On the other hand, garnishes usually consist of uncooked or lightly cooked scallions, parsley, and other vegetables; they have a lighter, more expansive quality. Condiments concentrate the energy and nutrients in dishes, while garnishes lighten it.

CONDIMENTS

Condiments can be purchased at natural foods stores or they can be made at home. They should be kept in tightly sealed containers or glass jars. Homemade condiments are fresher than store-bought varieties, and the ingredients can be specially balanced to suit your needs. The most frequently used varieties are listed below.

- **Gomashio**.   Among the regularly used condiments, gomashio (sesame salt) is especially nutritious. It is rich in calcium, iron, and other nutrients. It is an excellent source of polyunsaturated vegetable oil in its whole form. Also, because they are roasted, the sesame seeds in gomashio are easier to digest. The roasted sea salt in gomashio provides a harmonious balance to the oil in the seeds. A small amount can be used daily. Gomashio is especially delicious when freshly made and sprinkled on whole grain porridges in the morning. See page 152 for instructions on how to make gomashio.

The proportion of sesame seeds to sea salt in gomashio averages about 16 to 1. For children, who need much less salt than adults, a ratio of approximately 25 to 1 can be used. The best-quality sesame seeds for use in gomashio are natural black sesame seeds. It is important to be careful when choosing seeds, however, because some black seeds are dyed. To distinguish dyed seeds from natural ones, put them in water. If the seeds have been dyed, the artificial coloring will gradually dissolve and the water will turn black.

- **Sea-Vegetable Powders.**   These condiments are an excellent way to introduce mineral-rich sea vegetables into your breakfasts, and are quite delicious when sprinkled on whole grain porridges and other breakfast dishes. Those made from nori and dulse are the lightest-tasting and are rich in iron. Kombu and kelp powders are the richest-tasting, while wakame powders are characterized by a delicious, mild salty flavor. Sea-vegetable powders are prepared by roasting the sea vegetables for about 10–15 minutes, until dark and crisp. Next, they are crushed and ground in a suribachi until they become fine powder. They may be combined with roasted sesame seeds or used plain. Sea-vegetable powders can also be purchased in natural foods stores.

- **Toasted Nori Strips**.   Strips or squares of toasted nori are delicious when used as a garnish for porridge and breakfast soups. Nori contains about four times more vitamin A than carrots and ten times more than spinach. Additional information on nori and toasting instructions can be found on page 87.

- **Umeboshi Plums**.   Generally available in ready-to-eat form at most natural foods stores, umeboshi plums are also good for use at breakfast. They grow in the warmer southern and middle regions of Japan and are related to the apricot. Traditionally fermented with sea salt and shiso leaves, umeboshi plums have a sour, salty taste. They are a very well-balanced food, containing strong centering energy. They also have a wide range of uses. They are especially delicious when eaten with hot brown rice porridge in the morning. Their alkaline quality soothes and stimulates the stomach and the digestive organs.

- **Tekka**.   This is a traditional condiment made of burdock, carrots, lotus root, hatcho miso, and ginger that have been cooked down into a concentrated black powder. Tekka is recommended for use at breakfast. Since it provides very strong, concentrated energy, tekka is best used in small amounts when sprinkled on whole grain porridges and other dishes.

- **Seeds**.   Lightly roasted seeds can be sprinkled on morning porridges or other dishes for added taste and nutrients. Compared to meat and dairy products, seeds are a much better source of protein, and the fats and oils they contain are either neutral or unsaturated. However, their composition is not as balanced as that of whole grains. Seeds are higher in fat, higher in protein, and much lower in complex carbohydrates.

They are, however, very high in fiber, iron, calcium, and vitamins A, B, and E. Sesame and pumpkin seeds are especially rich in iron, containing about five times more than meat and more than any other plant foods, with the exception of sea vegetables. Sesame seeds are also a major source of calcium, containing about ten times that of a comparable amount of dairy milk.

- **Green Nori Flakes (Ao Nori).** Available, prepackaged, in most natural and macrobiotic foods stores, this particular type of nori is very delicious sprinkled over morning cereals. Green nori flakes are especially rich in iron and have a mild, bitter flavor.
- **Shiso Leaves.** These leaves are used in the process of making umeboshi plums. They are red, which is what gives the plums their color. The English name for shiso is the beefsteak plant. Shiso leaves have a tangy, salty-sour flavor. They help stimulate the appetite. Because of the salt they contain, they are best used in moderation. Raw shiso leaves may be minced and sprinkled over foods, minced and dry-roasted, or dry-roasted and ground into a fine powder. They are delicious when sprinkled on brown rice or other soft breakfast porridges.
- **Tamari Soy Sauce.** Tamari soy sauce (shoyu) is used more often as a seasoning than as a condiment. Occasionally, it may be used moderately, sprinkled over noodles or added to broths and tamari soy sauce-based soups. It is not recommended to add tamari soy sauce to miso soups, as this combination may cause cravings or overeating.

SWEETENERS

Natural sweeteners made from whole grains can also be used, on occasion, to sweeten porridges and other breakfast dishes. Some commonly used natural sweeteners are listed below.

- **Amazake (fermented rice milk).** Amazake is creamy, thick, and delicious when added to morning cereals. It is made from fermented sweet rice and a grain starter called koji. Amazake can also be served warm or chilled as a beverage. It can be used in making a variety of sugar-free natural desserts.
- **Barley Malt.** This sweetener is made by fermenting barley and then cooking down the resulting liquid. It has a rich toasted flavor, a dark opaque color, and a thick consistency. It can be used in making natural desserts or as an occasional sweetener in breakfast porridges. It is important to obtain the 100 percent variety, rather than barely malt that has been mixed with refined corn syrup.
- **Hato Mugi Malt.** Another occasionally used, natural sweetener is hato mugi malt. It is a delicious malt concentrate made from pearl barley and has a taste similar to butterscotch.

- **Rice Syrup**.   Rice syrup can be white, transparent, or amber in color and has a milder flavor and a more delicate texture than barley malt. It is usually made with a small amount of barley malt. The subtle flavor and light taste of rice syrup adds a wonderful sweetness to special-occasion foods like pancakes or waffles. Natural rice syrup can also be used, once in a while, to add sweetness to morning porridge.

These natural grain sweeteners are far more healthful than the artificial syrups sold commercially. Labels on these products are often misleading. A label may read "maple syrup," but will actually contain large amounts of refined sugar, water, artificial colorings, and a variety of chemicals. Tropical sweeteners, such as raw sugar cane, date sugar, chocolate, carob, and sorghum molasses, are best avoided by those in temperate climates. These products are high in fructose, glucose, or sucrose and can cause elevated blood sugar levels. Honey and genuine maple syrup also consist primarily of simple sugars and are best avoided for optimal health.

Gomashio

1 tablespoon sea salt
1 cup tan or black sesame seeds

Yield: Approximately 1/2 cup

Heat up a dry skillet. Add the sea salt and dry-roast until the color changes from white to an off-white or ivory color. Place the roasted sea salt in a suribachi and grind to a very fine powder. Wash the sesame seeds, place in a strainer, and drain. Heat up a skillet, and place the drained, damp sesame seeds in. Dry-roast, stirring constantly, until most of the moisture evaporates from the seeds and they begin to pop. Reduce the flame to medium-low and continue to roast, stirring constantly to cook evenly and to prevent burning. Fill a dry tablespoon with sesame seeds from the skillet, then pour them back in. If the seeds are done, they will not stick to the tablespoon. If any of the seeds still stick to the spoon, they are not completely roasted and moisture still remains in the seeds. Continue roasting until no seeds stick to the tablespoon. When they are thoroughly roasted, remove the seeds and place in the suribachi along with the finely ground sea salt. Grind slowly in a circular motion, applying constant pressure with the wooden pestle until the seeds are about 80 percent crushed. Allow to cool completely. To store, place in a tightly sealed glass jar until ready to use. This will keep about one week. Sprinkle lightly on grains, noodles, or vegetables.

Skillet-Roasted Kombu Powder

5 strips kombu, 10–12 inches long

Yield: Approximately 1/2 cup

Heat a cast iron skillet on a high flame. Break the kombu strips in half and place them, unwashed, in the heated skillet. Cover and reduce the flame to low. Dry-roast until the kombu becomes very brittle and crumbles easily in your hands. While roasting, constantly turn the kombu over and move it around in the skillet to prevent burning. This process will take approximately 30 minutes. After roasting, remove the kombu, place in a suribachi, and grind to a very fine powder. Allow to cool completely, then place in a tightly sealed glass jar for storage. To use, sprinkle sparingly on grains, noodles, or vegetables.

Miso-Scallion Condiment

4–5 medium-sized scallions with roots
1 1/2 teaspoons dark sesame oil
2–3 tablespoons puréed barley miso
2–3 tablespoons water

Yield: Approximately 1/2 cup

Wash the scallions and their roots. Finely mince the scallion roots and place on a plate. Slice the green portion of the scallions into 1/4-inch-thick slices. Heat the sesame oil in a cast iron or stainless steel skillet. Add the scallion roots and sauté for about 1 minute. Add the scallions, but do not sauté. Push the scallions toward the edge of the skillet, forming a small hole in the center. Pour the water and the puréed miso into the hole. Cover, bring to a boil, reduce the flame to medium-low, and simmer about 5–7 minutes. Mix well before placing in a serving bowl. A small amount of *Miso-Scallion Condiment* can be eaten on the side with breakfast dishes once a week or so. It is very strong and should be used in moderation. Instead of scallions, try chives or leeks, using the same proportions as above.

Oven-Roasted Kombu Powder

5 strips kombu, 10–12 inches long

Yield: Approximately 1/2 cup

Place the unwashed kombu on a baking sheet and place in the oven at 350° F. Bake for about 20 minutes or until crispy and easy to crush. Be careful not to burn. The color should be a brownish-green, not blackish-green. Remove the kombu, place in a suribachi, and grind to a very fine powder. Store in a tightly sealed glass jar and use sparingly on grain, noodle, or vegetable dishes.

Wakame Powder

5 strips wakame, 10–12 inches long

Yield: Approximately 1/2 cup

Place the unwashed wakame on a baking sheet and place in a 350° F oven for 20 minutes or until dark and crisp, but not charred. Remove and place in a suribachi. Grind to a very fine powder. Store in a tightly sealed glass jar. Sprinkle on grain, noodle, or vegetable dishes.

Goma-Wakame Powder

1/2 cup tan or white sesame seeds
5 strips wakame, 10–12 inches long

Yield: Approximately 3/4 cup

Place the unwashed wakame on a baking sheet and roast in a 350° F oven for 20 minutes until dark and crisp, but not charred. While the wakame is roasting, wash, rinse, and drain the sesame seeds. Dry-roast in a stainless steel skillet, the same as for making *Gomashio* (page 152). Remove the wakame, place in a suribachi, and grind to a very fine powder. Then add the roasted sesame seeds and grind until the seeds are about 80 percent crushed. Allow to cool. Store in a tightly sealed glass jar and use as a condiment on grains, noodles, or vegetables.

For a variation, combine roasted kombu or dulse with sesame seeds for a different flavor. Use as above.

Shio Kombu

2 strips kombu, 10–12 inches long
1 1/4 cups water
1/3–1/2 cup tamari soy sauce

Yield: Approximately 1/3 cup

Place the kombu in a bowl, cover with cold water, and soak for 3–5 minutes until soft enough to slice. Remove the kombu, reserving the soaking water. Slice the kombu into 1-inch squares and place in a saucepan. Cover with water (including the soaking water) and the tamari soy sauce. Cover the saucepan, bring to a boil, and reduce the flame to medium-low. Simmer for about 45–60 minutes until nearly all the liquid has evaporated. Remove the kombu and place in a small serving bowl. This is very salty and should be eaten in moderation. To store, place in a glass jar and keep in the refrigerator. Shio kombu will keep several months.

For a milder version, use 1 1/4 cups of water and 1/4 cup tamari soy sauce. You may also add 1–2 tablespoons of ginger that has been sliced into very thin matchsticks. The ginger should be added at the beginning of cooking. For another variation, add, at the beginning, 1 tablespoon of ginger matchsticks and 2–3 tablespoons of dried sardines (chirimen or chuba). Dry-roast the sardines several minutes before cooking with the kombu. For a sweeter variation, try adding a little brown rice syrup or barley malt to the kombu during the last 1–2 minutes of cooking. Toasted tan sesame seeds may also be added at the end of cooking to any of the variations mentioned.

Shio Nori

1 package untoasted nori (10 sheets)
1 1/2–2 cups water
Tamari soy sauce

Yield: Approximately 1 1/2 cup

Tear the nori into small pieces (about 1-inch squares) then place in a saucepan. Add the water and bring to a boil. Reduce the flame to medium-low, cover the saucepan, and simmer for 20 minutes. Add several drops of the tamari soy sauce for a mild salty taste or up to 2 tablespoons for a saltier flavor. Cover and simmer another 5–10 minutes or until most of the liquid has evaporated and the nori becomes a thick paste. Remove and place in a small serving bowl. Shio nori should be eaten in small amounts along with grains, noodles, or vegetable dishes. To store, allow to cool completely before placing in a tightly sealed glass jar. Refrigerate. Shio nori that has been prepared with a small amount of tamari soy sauce will keep for several days; if more soy sauce was used in its preparation, it will keep for up to two weeks.

Wakame-Sesame Seed Condiment

1 cup wakame, soaked and sliced into 1-inch lengths
1 1/2 tablespoons brown rice or sweet brown rice vinegar
1 1/2 tablespoons tamari soy sauce
1/4 cup water
2 tablespoons tan sesame seeds, roasted
(see page 50 for roasting instructions)

Yield: Approximately 1 1/4 cup

Place the wakame in a saucepan. Add the vinegar, tamari soy sauce, and water. Bring to a boil, cover the saucepan, and reduce the flame to medium-low. Simmer for about 15–20 minutes or until almost all of the liquid has evaporated. Mix in the roasted sesame seeds and place in a serving bowl. This condiment can be sprinkled on breakfast porridge or other dishes from time to time.

Green Pepper, Onion, and Miso Condiment

Dark sesame oil
1 medium onion, diced
1 green pepper, diced or sliced into long strips
1/4 cup water
3 tablespoons puréed barley miso

Yield: Approximately 1 cup

Brush a small amount of oil in a skillet and heat up. Add the onions and sauté for 1 minute. Next, add the green pepper and sauté for 1–2 minutes. Push the onions and green peppers toward the edge of the skillet to form a small hole in the center. Pour the water and puréed miso into the hole. Cover and cook for 10 minutes on a medium-low flame until the onions an peppers are tender and sweet. Mix and place in a serving bowl. This dish is salty, so use it moderately. It is quite delicious served over udon or somen. For a change, try using minced parsley or carrot tops instead of peppers and onions.

Shiso-Sesame Condiment

1/4 cup dried shiso leaf condiment (prepackaged)
1/2 cup tan sesame seeds, roasted (see page 50 for roasting instructions)
1/4 cup green nori flakes

Yield: Approximately 1 cup

Place the shiso leaf condiment in a suribachi and grind to a fine powder. Add the roasted sesame seeds and grind until about half-crushed. Add the green nori flakes and grind several seconds. Place in a tightly sealed glass container to store. Sprinkle small amounts on grains, noodles, or vegetables.

Parsley-Pumpkin Seed Condiment

1/2 cup pumpkin seeds, roasted (see page 50 for roasting instructions)
1 cup parsley, finely minced
Water
Tamari soy sauce

Yield: Approximately 1 cup

Finely chop the roasted pumpkin seeds on a cutting board. Next, place the seeds in a suribachi and grind 2–3 minutes. Place enough water in a skillet to just cover the bottom. Add the chopped parsley, cover, and bring to a boil. Reduce the flame to medium-low and sprinkle several drops of tamari soy sauce over the parsley for a mild salty flavor. Cover and simmer for about 1–2 minutes. Remove the parsley and place it in the suribachi with the ground pumpkin seeds. Mix together and place in a serving dish. A teaspoonful or two can be sprinkled on breakfast porridge or other dishes several times per week. For a different flavor, try using sunflower or tan sesame seeds.

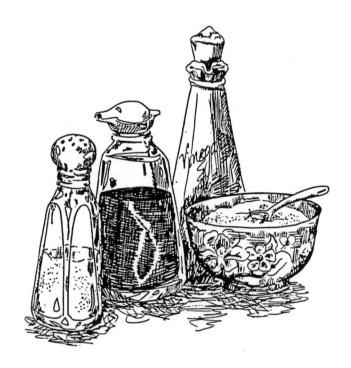

Chapter Nine

CAFFEINE-FREE BEVERAGES

Caffeine is powerfully charged with yin, expansive energy. Coffee, for example, causes the body's energy to move upward toward the head, stimulating the front part of the brain and facilitating mental activity. The downside to coffee is that it weakens us physically, and can lead to chronic fatigue, digestive upset, nervousness, and sexual dysfunction. It also counteracts the downward energy that helps us relax and fall asleep at night. Coffee is, therefore, a leading cause of the inability to sleep well, especially when taken in the evening.

People turn to coffee, soft drinks, and other caffeinated beverages in the morning because they have trouble generating active upward energy. The main reason for this is the chronic overconsumption of strongly contractive foods high in saturated fat, especially meat, cheese and other dairy products, eggs, and poultry. These foods create stagnation in the body and block the flow of energy. When someone develops this condition, they often use coffee, soda, other caffeinated beverages, and simple sugars (including those in frozen orange juice) to "jolt" their energy into functioning and to temporarily break through stagnation. However, this sudden high is quickly followed by a low, at which time another jolt becomes necessary. The body then becomes dependent on this outside push, setting up a cycle of addiction and dependency. The end result is an almost constant need to be stimulated in this way.

RECOMMENDED BEVERAGES

Eating a naturally balanced diet can help us break free from these cycles and establish natural balance. The beverages that we recommend for breakfast are natural and caffeine-free. They also contain no chemical additives or refined sugar, and are derived from plants that are native to the temperate zones (unlike coffee and tropical fruit drinks), thus making it easier to maintain harmony with the immediate environment. Some of the more popular macrobiotic breakfast drinks are discussed below, as well as guidelines for their preparation and use.

- **Bancha Tea.**   This is the most frequently consumed beverage at macrobiotic breakfasts. It is picked in midsummer from the large and mature leaves, stems, and twigs of the bancha tea bush. These are called, respectively, bancha leaf tea, bancha stem tea, and bancha twig tea. Traditionally picked by hand in the high mountains of Asia, the bancha leaves, stems, and twigs are roasted and cooled up to four separate times in large iron cauldrons. This procedure, as well as the late harvest when the caffeine has naturally receded from the tea bush, creates a tea containing virtually no caffeine or tannin, especially in the stem and twig parts. Also, unlike other teas, which are acidic, bancha is slightly alkaline and thus has a soothing, beneficial effect on digestion, blood quality, and the mind. It doesn't block, nor does it hyperstimulate, the smooth flow of upward energy in the morning. Bancha twig tea is also known as *kukicha* tea, from the Japanese term for "twig tea."

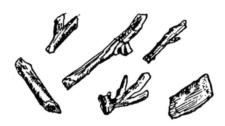

Bancha twigs and stems

- **Cereal Grain Tea.**   A delicious morning beverage can be made by roasting whole cereal grains and preparing them in the same way as ordinary tea. Roasted barley tea, or *mugicha* as it is known in Japan, is very soothing to the body and is quite appropriate in the morning. Roasted brown rice tea has a unique nutty flavor and can also be enjoyed at breakfast. Other grain teas, such as millet tea, oat tea, and buckwheat tea, may also be made in this way. All whole grain teas are suitable for daily use at breakfast or other meals. For variety, they may be mixed with bancha tea in various proportions.

- **Cereal Grain Coffee.** These coffees, made from roasted grains, beans, and chicory, can be enjoyed at breakfast. They provide a nourishing alternative to regular coffee or decaffeinated coffee, which is usually processed with chemicals. Grain coffee can be prepared at home or purchased in natural foods stores. Those made with 100 percent cereal grains, wild grasses, beans, and other vegetable-quality ingredients, and those containing no honey, molasses, or other strong sweeteners and fruit powders are suitable for occasional use.
- **Juice.** Juice made from fresh fruits or vegetables can be enjoyed on special occasions at breakfast by those in normal good health. However, since juice is a very concentrated product, it should be used sparingly and in small amounts. Unprocessed apple juice or apple cider, made from pressed organic apples and not from concentrate, is the most balanced of all fruit juices. Other temperate-climate fruit juices such as grape, pear, apricot, and cranberry juice may also be enjoyed from time to time. For those living in the temperate zones, orange, grapefruit, papaya, and other tropical or semitropical fruit juices are not recommended for optimal health, especially when they are made from concentrate.
- **Soymilk.** This beverage has traditionally been enjoyed in the Far East and is becoming increasingly popular in America and Europe. Several naturally processed soymilks are now available in natural foods stores. Those containing pearl barley, barley malt, and other grain or vegetable-quality ingredients, as well as a small amount of sea salt or kombu as a mineral source, are better for health than those containing honey, carob, chocolate, or other strong sweeteners. Because of its concentrated nature, soymilk is recommended only occasionally and in small amounts. Amazake (sweet rice milk) is preferable for use on breakfast porridges, puffed whole grain cereals, or as an occasional morning beverage.

High-Quality Drinking Water

A source of natural, high-quality water is essential for daily cooking and drinking. Natural spring or well water that is moving and alive (charged with natural energy from the earth) is best. City tap water often contains chlorine, as well as pesticide residues, detergents, nitrates, and heavy metals such as lead. Several mechanical methods are used to filter tap water of impurities, but it is still preferable to drink natural spring water that comes up from the earth or clear well water from an underground vein. However, it is important to have spring or well water tested before using it to make sure it is safe. Ordinary tap water can be used for washing your foods and utensils.

Bancha Tea

1 tablespoon bancha twigs
1 quart water

Yield: 1 quart

For a stronger beverage, first place the twigs in a dry stainless steel skillet and roast them for several minutes. For a lighter tea, simply place the twigs in a teakettle without roasting. Add the water and place the kettle over a high flame. Bring to a boil, then reduce the flame to low. For a mild tea, simmer 2–3 minutes; a stronger tea requires simmering the twigs for 10 minutes. Serve hot.

Brown Rice Tea

1/2 cup uncooked brown rice
1 quart water

Yield: 1 quart

Place the washed rice in a dry, heated skillet and roast until it turns golden brown, stirring constantly to evenly roast and prevent burning. Remove the rice and place in a teakettle with 1 quart of water. Bring the water to boil, reduce the flame to low, and simmer for approximately 15–20 minutes. Strain through a tea strainer and serve hot.

As a variation, try other grains such as barley or hato mugi (unroasted pearl barley), or combine roasted rice with a small amount of bancha twigs. Tea made from brown rice and barley is also very refreshing in the morning or any time of day.

Barley Tea

Prepackaged, roasted, unhulled barley for making tea can be found in most natural foods stores. It is sometimes sold under the name mugicha.

1 tablespoon roasted barley
1 quart water

Yield: 1 quart

Roast the barley in a dry skillet over a low flame until it turns golden brown. Stir constantly to evenly roast the barley and prevent burning. Place the roasted barley in a kettle filled with 1 quart of water. Bring the water to a boil, reduce the flame to low, and simmer to desired strength. For a mild tea, simmer for 3–5 minutes. Simmer 10–15 minutes for a stronger tea. In the summer months this tea is very refreshing when slightly chilled and served with a slice of lemon.

Brown Rice and Bancha Tea

1 tablespoon bancha twigs
1/4 cup uncooked brown rice
1 quart water

Yield: 1 quart

Dry roast the rice as instructed in *Brown Rice Tea*, page 162. Place all ingredients in a kettle and bring to a boil. Reduce the flame to low and simmer about 10 minutes. Strain the tea through a bamboo tea strainer and serve.

Ready-Made Grain Coffee

1 teaspoon grain coffee
1 cup boiling water

Place a teaspoonful of grain coffee in a cup and pour boiling water over it. Stir and drink.

Homemade Grain Coffee

3 cups uncooked brown rice
2 1/2 cups winter wheat
1 1/2 cups azuki beans
2 cups chickpeas
1 cup chicory root

Yield: Approximately 4 ounces

Separately dry-roast each ingredient in a skillet until dark in color (see page 50 for roasting instructions). Mix all of the roasted grains, beans, and chicory together and grind to a fine powder in a grain mill. Brew coffee using 1 teaspoonful of the powder per cup of water. If left to boil, the grain coffee tends to foam, so quickly reduce the heat and simmer for 5–10 minutes. Store the powder in an airtight container.

Homemade Amazake

4 cups uncooked sweet brown rice
8 cups spring water
1/2 cup koji

Yield: Approximately 2 quarts

Wash the rice, drain, and soak in the water overnight. Place rice and soaking water in a pressure cooker and bring up to pressure. Lower heat and cook for 45 minutes. When cool enough to handle, mix the koji into the rice with your hands. Transfer the mixture to a glass bowl (do not use metal), cover with a wet cloth or towel, and place near an oven, radiator, or any other warm place. Allow to ferment 4–8 hours. During the fermentation period, occasionally stir the mixture to melt the koji.

After fermenting, put the amazake in a pot and bring to a boil. When bubbles appear, turn off the heat and allow the mixture to cool. Refrigerate in a tightly sealed glass bowl or jar. When fermentation has stopped, it will keep for a couple of weeks.

To serve as a breakfast drink, first stir the amazake, then put it in a saucepan with a pinch of sea salt and enough spring water to achieve the desired consistency. Bring to a boil and serve hot or allow to cool and serve chilled. Amazake can also be poured over bowls of puffed cereal (corn, rice, wheat, millet, etc.) or added to hot breakfast porridge for additional sweetness.

Sweet Vegetable Drink

1/2 cup onions, finely sliced
1/2 cup carrots, finely sliced
1/2 cup cabbage, finely sliced
1/2 cup squash, finely sliced
8 cups water

Yield: Approximately 1 quart

Place the sliced vegetables in a pot and add water. Cover the pot, bring to a boil, turn the flame to low, and simmer for 15–20 minutes. Pour the liquid through a fine mesh strainer into a large glass jar. The strained liquid—or sweet vegetable drink—can be stored for several days in the refrigerator. To serve this as a breakfast drink, heat in a saucepan until warm, or allow it to sit outside of the refrigerator until it reaches room temperature.

Chapter Ten

SPECIAL
BREAKFAST
DISHES

A wide variety of delicious and healthful breakfast treats can be made from the whole natural foods listed in Chapter Two. As with other foods in the macrobiotic diet, these dishes are cholesterol-free and very low in saturated fat. They contain no refined sugar or chemical additives and are made with all-natural ingredients.

Special-occasion breakfast dishes are traditionally prepared on Sunday mornings, when more time is available to make and enjoy them. They include dishes not normally eaten during the week. Of course, preparing these breakfast treats should be determined by individual desires and preferences.

Included in this chapter are such specialties as *Tofu French Toast, Mochi Waffles* and *Whole Wheat Crepes*, as well as a variety of fruit and vegetable fillings, tofu cheeses, dips, and spreads to complement them. Recipes for *Whole Wheat Bagels, Brown Rice Bread*, and *Unleavened Apple Muffins* are also included. Children will love the *Tofu MacroMuffins* and *Yeasted Whole Wheat Donuts*, as well as the *Yeasted Whole Wheat Cinnamon-Raisin Rolls*.

These dishes can be enjoyed from time to time by those in general good health. Persons who are adopting macrobiotics because of a health problem may need to wait until normal health is established before including some of these dishes into their diets. If you aren't sure about the appropriateness of any of the dishes in this chapter, please check with a macrobiotic teacher or educational center.

The special dishes presented in this chapter are delicious when incorporated in your breakfast menus along with soup, porridge, and other side dishes.

Tofu French Toast

1 cake firm-style tofu (16 ounces)
1/2 cup water
1 teaspoon tamari soy sauce
8 slices unyeasted sourdough bread
Dark sesame or corn oil

Yield: 8 slices

Place the tofu, water, and tamari soy sauce in a blender and blend to a creamy consistency. Heat a small amount of dark sesame or corn oil in a skillet. Pour the creamed tofu into a large bowl. Dip the slices of bread into the tofu mixture, lightly covering both sides. Fry the tofu-coated bread until golden brown, then remove and place on a serving platter. Repeat this process with the remaining ingredients. Top with any of the natural toppings found in this chapter and serve with soup or porridge and a cup of tea.

Sourdough Waffles

1 1/2 cups whole wheat pastry flour
1 cup whole wheat flour
2 tablespoons sesame oil
1/4 teaspoon sea salt
1 cup cooked soft rice
1 cup soured seitan starch water (see page 77)
1 cup cold water

Yield: 8–10 waffles

Combine all ingredients, mix well, and allow to sit overnight in a warm place. Use a large bowl to let the batter sit in, as it will ferment from the soured seitan water and rise. Oil a waffle iron and heat. Add batter and cook until golden brown, then add your favorite natural topping. Serve with other breakfast dishes.

Mochi Waffles

Mochi waffles are delicious as is or when added to miso soup. They can also be served with your favorite natural topping.

8 pieces of mochi, 2 ×3 × 1/4 inch

Yield: 8 waffles

Place one piece of mochi at a time in a heated waffle iron. Do not oil the iron. Cook until the mochi is crisp and slightly browned and does not stick to the waffle iron. Remove the waffle and repeat until all of the mochi has been used.

Buckwheat Pancakes

1 cup buckwheat flour
1 cup whole wheat pastry flour
1/8 teaspoon sea salt
1 1/2 cup apple juice or water
Dark sesame oil

Yields: 8–10 pancakes

Combine the dry ingredients. Gradually add apple juice or water to create the desired consistency for pancake batter. Mix very well with a fork or wire whisk or place in a blender, if necessary. Let the batter sit in a warm place overnight so that it begins to ferment. This will help the pancakes rise and become lighter when cooking.

Lightly oil a pancake griddle or skillet with dark sesame oil and heat up. Spoon a small amount of batter to form a round cake. Fry on one side until little air bubbles form on the surface. Flip over and fry the other side until golden brown. Remove and place on a serving platter. Add your favorite natural topping and serve with soup, porridge, or other side dishes.

Be careful about the height of the flame you use when cooking pancakes. If the flame is too high the pancakes might burn and if it is too low they will not cook thoroughly.

Apple-Raisin Topping

2 apples, cored and sliced
1 pear, cored and sliced
1/4 cup raisins
2 cups water or apple juice
Pinch of sea salt
2 tablespoons kuzu, diluted in 2–3 tablespoons water

Yield: 2 1/2–3 cups

Place the raisins, sea salt, and water or juice in a saucepan, and bring to a boil. Reduce the flame to low and simmer the raisins for about 5 minutes. Add the apples and pears. Cover and simmer the raisins and fruit slices over a medium-low flame for about 5 minutes until tender. Reduce the flame to low. Dilute the kuzu and add to the saucepan, stirring constantly to prevent lumping. Simmer several seconds until the kuzu thickens. The topping is now ready to pour over tofu French toast, pancakes, or waffles. Serve while hot.

Strawberry Topping

2 cups apple juice
Pinch of sea salt
1 pint fresh strawberries, washed, de-stemmed, and halved
2 teaspoons kuzu, diluted in 2–3 teaspoons water

Yield: 2 1/2–3 cups

Place the apple juice and sea salt in a saucepan. Bring to a boil. Reduce the flame to low, add the strawberries, and simmer for 2–3 minutes. Dilute the kuzu and add to the saucepan, stirring constantly to prevent lumping. When the sauce becomes thick and translucent, it is ready to serve over tofu French toast, pancakes, or waffles.

Lemon-Rice Syrup Topping

1/2 cup brown rice syrup
2 teaspoons freshly squeezed lemon juice
2–3 tablespoons water

Yield: 1/2 cup

Place the brown rice syrup and water in a saucepan. Heat up but do not boil. Reduce the flame to low, add the lemon juice, and mix in. Pour the hot syrup over tofu French toast, pancakes, or waffles.

Lemon-Kuzu-Rice Syrup Topping

1 cup apple juice
Pinch of sea salt
1/4 cup brown rice syrup
2 teaspoons freshly squeezed lemon juice
1 teaspoon kuzu, diluted in 1–2 teaspoons water

Yield: 1 1/4 cup

Place the apple juice, sea salt, and rice syrup in a saucepan and heat up. Reduce the flame to low. Dilute the kuzu and add to the saucepan, stirring constantly to prevent lumping. When thick, place the lemon juice in the saucepan and mix. The sauce is now ready to pour over tofu French toast, pancakes, or waffles.

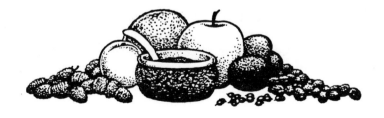

Barley Malt-Walnut Topping

1/2 cup barley malt
1/4 cup walnuts, roasted and chopped
2–3 tablespoons water

Yield: 3/4 cup

Heat the barley malt and water in a saucepan. Reduce the flame to low, add the walnuts, and mix. Remove from the flame. The topping is now ready to serve over tofu French toast, pancakes, or waffles.

Whole Wheat Crepes

2 cups whole wheat pastry flour
1/4 teaspoon sea salt
2 cups water

Yield: Approximately 9 crepes

Mix the flour and salt together in a bowl. Gradually add water to create a thin batter, stirring to remove lumps. For a lighter batter, blend in the blender or mix with an egg beater. Pour a small amount of batter onto a hot, oiled pancake griddle and smooth out with a spoon until the batter is very thin and round. This can be done by making a circular motion, very lightly and gently, on the batter with a spoon or soup ladle. Cook on one side until tiny bubbles appear on the surface. Flip the crepe over and fry the other side for about 1 minute. These cook quickly, so be careful not to burn them. Place your favorite fruit or vegetable filling on the crepe and roll up. Fasten with a toothpick, if necessary, and serve. The unfilled crepes can also be rolled up and served with the filling poured on top.

As a variation, buckwheat crepes can be made by using half pastry and half buckwheat flour. Slightly more water may be added when using buckwheat, as it absorbs water more readily than other flours.

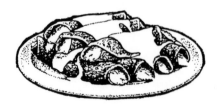

Vegetable Filling

Dark sesame oil
1/4 cup onions, sliced into thin half-moons
1/2 cup mushrooms, thinly sliced
1/4 cup green pepper, diced
2 tablespoons burdock, sliced into thin matchsticks
1/4 cup carrots, sliced into thin matchsticks
1/2 cup green cabbage, finely shredded
Water
Tamari soy sauce or sea salt

Yield: Approximately 1 1/2 cups

Heat a small amount of dark sesame oil in a skillet. Add the onions and sauté 1–2 minutes. Next, add the mushrooms and green peppers and sauté another 2–3 minutes. Finally, add the burdock, carrots, and cabbage. Place a small amount of water in the skillet so that it barely covers the bottom. Bring to a boil, cover, and reduce the flame to medium-low. Cook for several minutes until the vegetables are tender. Remove the cover and season with a little tamari soy sauce or sea salt. Continue to sauté until all of the liquid has evaporated. Place inside crepes and roll up.

Cherry Filling

2 cups cherries, pitted and halved
Water
Pinch of sea salt
3–4 teaspoons barley malt or rice syrup
1 heaping tablespoon kuzu, diluted in 2 tablespoons water

Yield: 1 1/2 cups

Place about 1/8 inch of water in a saucepan and add the cherries and sea salt. Add the barley malt or rice syrup to sweeten the cherries if necessary. Bring to a boil, cover, and reduce the flame to medium-low. Simmer until the cherries are soft. Reduce the flame to low and add a very small amount of diluted kuzu to thicken. Stir to prevent lumping. When thick, remove and place inside or on top of the crepes.

Any type of fruit, fresh or dried, can be used to make a filling for crepes. Dried fruit should first be soaked and then sliced before using.

Peach-Raisin Filling

2 cups (2 medium-sized) peaches, washed and sliced into
1/4–1/2-inch wedges
1/3 cup raisins
2 cups water
Small pinch of sea salt
1 heaping tablespoon kuzu, diluted in 2 tablespoons water
3–4 teaspoons brown rice syrup

Yield: 3 cups

Place the peaches in a saucepan with the raisins. Add two cups water and a pinch of sea salt. Cover the pot, turn the flame to high, and bring to a boil. Turn the flame to medium-low and simmer for 10 minutes. Add diluted kuzu and rice syrup to the peaches. Stir to prevent lumping and cook for about 1 minute.

   Place each crepe on a serving plate and spoon 2–3 tablespoons of filling over the center of each crepe. Then roll up and spoon 3–4 tablespoons of kuzu sauce on top. If peaches are out of season, the same topping can be made using fresh apples.

Tofu MacroMuffins

3–4 whole wheat English muffins
3–4 pieces of firm-style tofu, 1/4-inch-thick slices
Sauerkraut
Alfalfa sprouts
Lettuce

Yield: 3–4 muffin sandwiches

Slice the muffins in half and toast. Pan-fry the tofu as described in *Pan-Fried Tofu Slices*, page 138. Place a slice of tofu on the bottom half of each muffin. Put 1–2 teaspoons of sauerkraut on top of each tofu slice and garnish with lettuce and sprouts. Place the remaining half of the muffin on top. Serve for breakfast or wrap for lunch.

Yeasted Whole Wheat Bagels

1/2 tablespoon active dry yeast
1 1/4 cups warm water
1 tablespoon whole wheat pastry flour
1 1/2 cups whole wheat pastry flour
3 1/2–4 cups whole wheat bread flour
1/4 cup brown rice syrup
1/2 cup light sesame or corn oil
1 teaspoon sea salt

Yield: 10–12 bagels

Place the yeast and 1 tablespoon of whole wheat pastry flour in a cup and add 1/4 cup warm water. Mix until dissolved. Let the yeast sit for about 10 minutes.

Mix together 1 1/2 cups whole wheat bread flour, 1 1/2 cups whole wheat pastry flour, 1 cup warm water, 1/4 cup brown rice syrup, and the dissolved yeast mixture. Cover the bowl with a damp towel and let rise until it has doubled in size.

Once doubled, add the oil, sea salt, and the remaining 2–2 1/2 cups whole wheat bread flour. Form into a ball of dough, and knead for about 5–7 minutes. Cover the bowl with a damp towel and let it rise for about 1 hour in a warm place.

Next, press down the dough, cover with a damp towel, and let it rise again for another 20–25 minutes. After the final rising, take a handful of dough and roll it out into a 3/4-inch-thick strand, about 6–7 inches long, and connect the ends together. Repeat until all the dough is used up. As an alternative, the dough can also be cut with a doughnut cutter.

Take a pot of water and bring it to a boil. Place the dough rings in the boiling water for about 10 minutes. Remove the boiled dough and place on a lightly oiled cookie or baking sheet. Set in a warm place and let rise for another 20 minutes.

Preset your oven for 375° F and bake the bagels for about 25 minutes or until golden brown. Let them cool. Serve plain or with your favorite spread.

Whole Wheat Bagels with Tofu Cream Cheese

Whole wheat bagels can be bought pre-made, or you could try your hand at making your own (recipe found on page 175).

3–4 whole wheat bagels
3/4 cup tofu cream cheese (see page 178 for recipe)
1 small red onion, thinly sliced into rings
Alfalfa sprouts for garnish
3–6 thin dill pickle slices
3–4 lettuce leaves

Yield: 3–4 bagel sandwiches

Slice the bagels in half and leave as is or toast. Spread a 1/4-inch-thick layer of tofu cream cheese on each half. Garnish with thinly sliced red onion rings, a few sprouts, several pieces of dill pickle, and fresh lettuce. Place the top and bottom halves of the bagels together to form delicious breakfast sandwiches.

Tofu Cream Spread

Water (for blanching vegetables)
2 tablespoons onions, finely diced
2 tablespoons carrots, minced
2 tablespoons celery, minced
1 cake firm-style tofu (16 ounces)
1 tablespoon onion, grated
1 tablespoon scallions, finely chopped
3–4 tablespoons umeboshi vinegar
1/4 cup water
1 tablespoon organic tahini , roasted (see page 50 for roasting instructions)

Yield: Approximately 1 1/2 cups

Place a small amount of water in a saucepan and bring to a boil. To the boiling water add the diced onions, carrots, and celery; cook for 30 seconds, drain, and allow to cool.

Grind the roasted tahini in a suribachi until smooth. Next, using a hand food mill, purée the tofu directly into the suribachi. Mix well. Add the cooked vegetables to the suribachi along with the grated onion, scallions, umeboshi vinegar, and 1/4 cup of water. With a wooden pestle, purée all ingredients together until evenly mixed. Spread on whole wheat bagels, bread, crackers, or use as a dip with chips or raw vegetables (crudités).

Tofu Cheese

1 cake firm or extra-firm-style tofu (16 ounces)
Barley miso
Cotton cheesecloth

Yield: Approximately 1 cup

Place the tofu on a cutting board. Tilt the board over the edge of the sink, by propping it up with a book or dishcloth. Place a heavy object, such as a plate or another smaller cutting board, on top of the cake of tofu to apply slight pressure. This will allow water from the tofu to drain down the board and into the sink. Let drain for about 20–30 minutes.

Take the drained cake of tofu and cover it on all sides with a layer of clean, cotton cheesecloth. Completely encase the wrapped tofu in a 1/4-inch-thick layer of barley miso. Place the miso-coated tofu in a glass or ceramic bowl. Cover the bowl with a clean piece of cotton cheesecloth (to keep out any dust) and put in a warm place for 3–4 days (2–3 in warmer weather). During this time, the miso will be absorbed into the tofu and cause it to contract and slightly ferment.

Remove the miso-coated cheesecloth from the tofu, reserving the miso for future use in soups or vegetable dishes. Rinse the miso-pickled tofu under cold water to remove any leftover miso from its surface. Place on a cutting board and slice in the same manner as you would regular cheese. Serve on bagels, bread, or crackers.

As a variation, tamari soy sauce or umeboshi vinegar (or plums) may be sprinkled over the cake of tofu. Allow to sit several days before serving.

For a creamy tofu cheese spread, add 1/4 cup chopped scallions and 1/2 cup water to the tofu cheese (above) and purée till smooth and creamy. Use as a spread on bagels, bread, or crackers.

Tofu Cream Cheese

1 cake fresh, firm-style tofu (16 ounces)
1 tablespoon onion, finely grated
1 tablespoon umeboshi vinegar
Chopped scallions for garnish

Yield: Approximately 1 1/4 cup

Place the tofu in a hand food mill and grind. Add the umeboshi vinegar and grated onion. Mix well. Place the tofu cream in a serving dish and garnish with chopped scallions. Serve on toast, steamed bread, whole wheat English muffins, or crackers. This can also be used in whole grain bread sandwiches with lettuce and sprouts. Tofu cream cheese is also delicious as a dip for boiled, steamed, or raw vegetables.

Brown Rice Bread

4 cups whole wheat bread flour
1/4 teaspoon sea salt
4 cups cooked brown rice (let rice sit for 2 days and become slightly sour)
1/4 cup light sesame oil (optional)
Water
Pastry flour

Yield: 2 loaves

Mix together the whole wheat bread flour and sea salt. Add the brown rice and mix by sifting together with your hands. Add the oil (optional), and sift again. Next, add enough water to form a ball of dough. Knead the dough about 15 minutes (300–350 times). While you are kneading the dough, it will occasionally become sticky and difficult to knead. When this starts to happen, sprinkle a small amount of pastry flour on the sides and bottom of the bowl. Then proceed with the kneading again. The flour will prevent sticking and will make the dough firmer and easier to knead. It may be necessary to sprinkle pastry flour in the bowl several times during the kneading process.

Lightly oil two bread pans with light sesame oil and evenly coat them with a little whole wheat pastry flour. Divide the dough in half and form both halves into two loaves. Place the loaves in the bread pans. Gently press the dough down along the edges of the pans to create a slightly rounded effect. Then, with a knife, make a shallow, lengthwise slit about 1/4 inch deep, down the center of each loaf.

Take two clean kitchen towels dampened with warm water, and place one over each bread pan. Place the covered pans in a warm place and allow the loaves to rise for 8–12 hours. When the towels become dry, dampen again with warm water and place back over the dough. This may need to be done several times during the rising for optimum results.

After the dough has risen, place the loaves in a preheated, 300° F oven. After 15–20 minutes, raise the temperature to 350° F and continue to bake for approximately 1 hour and 10 minutes or until the loaves are golden brown. When the bread is done, remove from the pans and allow to cool on a wire rack. To store, place in brown paper bags and keep in the cupboard or refrigerator.

As a variation, after kneading the dough about 100 times, 2 cups of raisins can be added to this recipe to create loaves of delicious *Brown Rice-Raisin Bread*.

NOTE: For maximum results, it is best if the rice used is 2–3 days old and slightly sour. This causes the dough to rise much better. Bread also rises better if the dough is made early in the morning, is allowed to rise all day, and is baked in the evening.

Steamed Bread

Several slices unyeasted whole wheat or sourdough bread
Water

Place a steamer basket inside a pot and add 1/2 inch of water. Cover, place on a high flame, and bring to a boil. Remove the cover and place the bread slices in the steamer basket. Cover the pot again and steam 2–4 minutes (depending on how old the bread is) until soft and moist. Remove and place the slices of bread on a platter. Serve with any of the spreads or butters found in this chapter or with any of your favorite jams or jellies.

Miso-Tahini Spread

6 tablespoons organic tahini, roasted (see page 50
for roasting instructions)
1 tablespoon barley (mugi) miso
2–3 tablespoons scallions, finely chopped
1 tablespoon water

Yield: Approximately 1/2 cup

After roasting the tahini in a skillet, add the miso, chopped scallions, and water. Mix thoroughly and roast on a medium-low flame for 1–2 minutes. Remove from the flame. Place the *Miso-Tahini Spread* in a bowl. Spread very lightly (this is a little salty) on fresh, toasted, or steamed bread. It is also good on whole grain crackers.

Try adding chopped chives instead of scallions, or use other types of miso such as brown rice or mellow barley for a different flavor. Instead of tahini, try using sesame butter or peanut butter for variety.

Onion Butter

Dark sesame oil
10 medium onions, finely diced
Pinch of sea salt
Water

Yield: Approximately 2 cups

Place a small amount of dark sesame oil in a heavy pot and heat up. Add the onions and a small pinch of sea salt. Sauté the onions, stirring constantly, for 3–5 minutes until the onions are translucent. Add enough water to just cover the onions. Bring to a boil, reduce the flame to low, and simmer several hours until the onions become dark brown in color and very sweet in flavor. Occasionally during the cooking process, you may need to add small amounts of water to prevent burning. When the onion butter is done, allow to cool completely before placing it in a tightly sealed jar and refrigerating. Use immediately or store as above.

Instead of using onions, finely chopped carrots, squash, apples, or other fruits and vegetables may be used. To avoid the use of oil, the water-sautéing method may be used instead. At the end of cooking, tamari soy sauce or puréed miso can be used for a different flavor.

Corn Bread

3 cups cornmeal
1 cup whole wheat pastry flour
1/4 teaspoon sea salt
2 cups cooked brown rice
2 tablespoons corn oil
1 cup fresh sweet corn (optional depending on season)
2 1/2–3 cups water
Sesame oil

Serves: 4–6

In a mixing bowl, combine the cornmeal, pastry flour, and sea salt. Mix well. Add the cooked brown rice and mix together. Next, add the corn oil and the sweet corn, mixing thoroughly. Add the water and mix again.

Preheat the oven to 350° F. Lightly oil an 11 × 7 × 2-inch baking pan with a small amount of light sesame oil. Place the pan in the oven and heat the oil for about 3–5 minutes. Remove the pan, add the batter, and return to the oven. Bake for about 1 hour and 45 minutes until golden brown.

Unleavened Apple Muffins

2 cups whole wheat pastry flour
1 cup whole wheat bread flour
1/4 teaspoon sea salt
1/4 teaspoon cinnamon
3–4 tablespoons corn oil
1 3/4 cups apple juice
3 apples, peeled and diced

Yield: 12 muffins

Combine all dry ingredients in a mixing bowl. Add the oil and mix thoroughly. Next, mix in the apple juice. Add the apples to the batter and mix evenly. Preheat the oven to 350° F. Fill lightly oiled muffin cups to the top with batter. Bake 25–30 minutes or until golden brown.

For a lighter muffin, place the batter in a glass bowl, cover with a damp towel, and let sit in a warm place overnight. Then fill the muffin cups about 3/4 full and bake the same as above.

Unleavened Brown Rice Muffins

2 cups whole wheat bread flour
1 cup brown rice flour
1 cup cornmeal
1/4 teaspoon sea salt
3 1/2–4 tablespoons corn oil
1 cup soft-cooked brown rice cereal
3 cups water
1 cup raisins

Yield: 12 muffins

Combine all dry ingredients. Add the oil and mix well. Next, add the rice and mix. Finally, add the raisins and water and mix again. Preheat the oven to 325° F. Fill lightly oiled muffin cups to the top with batter. Bake for 25–30 minutes or until golden brown.

For a lighter muffin, allow the batter to sit overnight in a glass bowl covered with a damp towel. Then fill the muffin tins 3/4 full and bake as above.

Yeasted Whole Wheat Donuts

1/2 tablespoon active dry yeast
1 1/4 cups warm water
1 tablespoon whole wheat bread flour
1 3/4 cups whole wheat bread flour
1 1/2 cups whole wheat pastry flour
1 teaspoon sea salt
1/3 teaspoon cinnamon
1 1/2 tablespoons light sesame or corn oil
1 cup raisins

Yield: Approximately 12 donuts

Place the dry yeast and 1/4 cup of warm water in a cup, dissolve, and let sit for about 5 minutes. Mix in 1 tablespoon whole wheat bread flour and let sit for another 5–10 minutes. Combine the remaining whole wheat bread flour, pastry flour, sea salt, and cinnamon in a bowl. Add the oil and mix well. Next, mix in the raisins.

Gradually combine the yeast and the remaining cup of water with the flour mixture. Form into a ball of dough and knead for about 5–7 minutes. Place the dough in an oiled bowl, cover with a warm, damp towel, and let rise for about 4 hours in a warm place. The dough should double in size. Punch the dough down with your hands, cover with a damp towel, and let rise for another hour or so. Punch the dough down again, and roll out onto a floured surface, the same as if making pie crust. The dough should be about 1/3 inch thick. Cut out the donuts with a donut cutter.

Deep-fry the donuts for about 1 1/2–2 minutes or until slightly brown. Remove, place on paper towels or a draining rack, and allow to cool before eating.

Yeasted Whole Wheat Cinnamon-Raisin Rolls

1/2 tablespoon active dry yeast
1 1/4 cup warm water
1 tablespoon whole wheat bread flour
1 3/4 cups whole wheat bread flour
1 1/2 cups whole wheat pastry flour
1 teaspoon sea salt
1 1/2 tablespoons light sesame or corn oil

CINNAMON-RAISIN FILLING

2 cups raisins
1 cup apple juice
Barley malt
Cinnamon
2 cups walnuts, chopped and roasted
(see page 50 for roasting instructions)

Yield: Approximately 12 rolls

Follow the recipe instructions for *Yeasted Whole Wheat Donuts* (page 182) in preparing the pastry part of this recipe. About 1 hour before the dough is ready, soak the raisins in the apple juice. Remove the raisins and squeeze out any liquid.

Divide the dough in half and roll out onto a floured surface until the dough is 1/4–1/3 inch thick. Spread barley malt over the entire surface of the rolled-out dough. Sprinkle a little cinnamon over the barley malt. With your hands, mix the barley malt and cinnamon until it is evenly spread over the dough. Sprinkle half of the raisins and walnuts over the entire surface of the dough. Roll up the dough and pinch the ends together to seal. Slice the roll into 1–1 1/2-inch-thick rounds. Place the rolls, cut side up, on a lightly oiled baking sheet. Repeat the above process with the remaining half of the dough. In a preheated, 350° F oven, bake for 20–25 minutes until golden brown. Remove and place on a serving platter.

Sautéed Okara and Vegetables

Okara is soybean pulp, a by-product of tofu. It is best if used immediately after making fresh tofu, as it has a tendency to spoil easily. Okara is recommended for those in general good health.

Dark sesame oil
1/4 cup burdock, cut into thin matchsticks
2 shiitake mushrooms, soaked, de-stemmed, and thinly sliced
1/4 cup celery, sliced into thin diagonals
1/2 cup carrots, sliced into thin matchsticks
1/4 cup green beans, sliced into very thin diagonals
2 cups fresh okara
Water
Tamari soy sauce
1/4 cup roasted almonds, slivered or finely chopped
1/8 cup scallions or chives, finely chopped

Serves: 4

Heat a small amount of dark sesame oil in a skillet. Add the burdock and sauté for 2–3 minutes. Next, add the mushrooms and sauté for 1–2 minutes. Add the celery, carrots, and green beans. Sauté for 2–3 minutes. Add the okara, a small amount at a time, and mix in thoroughly with the vegetables. Sauté several minutes. If dry, add 1/4 cup of water while sautéing. Add several drops of tamari soy sauce, the almonds, and the chopped scallions. Mix well, cover, and simmer over a low flame for 2–3 minutes. Remove the cover and place in a serving bowl.

Scrambled Tofu with Mushrooms and Green Peppers

Dark sesame oil
1/2 cup onions, diced
1/2 cup mushrooms, thinly sliced
1/2 cup green pepper, thinly sliced (no seeds)
1/2 cup carrots, sliced into thin matchsticks
1 cake firm-style tofu (16 ounces)
Tamari soy sauce

Serves: 4

Heat a small amount of dark sesame oil in a skillet. Add the onions and sauté for 1–2 minutes. Next, sauté the mushrooms and green peppers for 2–3 minutes. Add the carrots, but do not sauté. Using your hands, crumble the tofu over the vegetables. Reduce the flame to medium-low, cover, and simmer several minutes until the vegetables are tender and the tofu becomes light and fluffy. Season lightly with tamari soy sauce. Cover and cook for another 3–5 minutes. Mix the ingredients together and place in a serving bowl. Serve with toast or steamed bread.

Summer Scrambled Tofu and Sweet Corn

Dark sesame oil
2–3 cups fresh sweet corn, removed from cob
1 cake firm-style tofu (16 ounces)
Umeboshi vinegar
1/2 cup scallions, chopped

Serves: 4

Lightly brush a small amount of oil in a skillet and heat up. Add the sweet corn and sauté for 1 minute. With your hands, crumble the tofu over the corn. Cover the skillet, reduce the flame to medium-low, and simmer until the corn is tender and the tofu is light and fluffy. Sprinkle several drops of umeboshi vinegar over the tofu. Add the scallions, but do not mix in. Cover the skillet and simmer for another 3–5 minutes. Mix thoroughly and place in a serving bowl.

Mochi and Vegetable Pancakes

Dark sesame oil
1/4 cup onion, diced
1/4 cup mushrooms, thinly sliced
1/4 cup carrots, sliced into thin matchsticks
1/2 cup cabbage or Chinese cabbage, finely shredded
Water
1/2 pound plain mochi, coarsely grated
1/2 sheet nori, toasted and cut into thin strips (see page 87)
Tamari soy sauce

Yield: 6–8 pancakes

Heat a small amount of oil in a skillet. Sauté the onions and mushrooms for 1–2 minutes. Next, add the carrots and cabbage and sauté 1 minute. Add enough water to just coat the bottom of the skillet. Cover, reduce the flame to low, and simmer for 3–4 minutes until the vegetables are tender. Remove the cover, sprinkle a few drops of tamari soy sauce on the vegetables, mix, and cook 1 minute more. Remove the vegetables and place in a bowl.

On a heated, dry pancake griddle, place 1/8–1/4 cup of mochi at a time in little mounds. Keep each mound of grated mochi separate. On top of each mound, place 1–2 tablespoons of the sautéed vegetables and a few strips of toasted nori. Next, quickly sprinkle a little more grated mochi on top of the vegetables to create a sandwich effect. Cook on each side until slightly browned. The mochi will melt, completely encasing the vegetables, and will puff up slightly. Remove and place on a serving platter. Repeat the above process until all of the ingredients have been used.

For a delicious change, instead of using sautéed vegetables, try adding your favorite fruit topping or sugar-free jam, jelly, or apple butter.

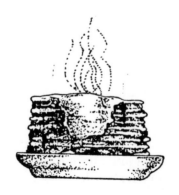

Glossary

Agar-agar. A white gelatin derived from a sea-vegetable, used in making aspics.

Amazake. A sweetener or refreshing drink made from sweet rice and koji starter that is allowed to ferment into a thick liquid. Hot amazake is a delicious sweet beverage. It may be referred to as amazake or amasake.

Arrowroot. A starch flour processed from the root of an American native plant. It is used as a thickening agent, similar to cornstarch or *kuzu*, for making sauces, stews, gravies, and desserts.

Azuki Bean. A small, dark red bean imported from Japan, but also grown in the United States. Good when cooked with *kombu** sea-vegetable. This bean may also be referred to as aduki or adzuki.

Bancha Tea. Correctly named kukicha, bancha tea is made by steeping the stems and leaves from mature Japanese tea bushes. This tea aids in digestion and contains no chemical dyes. Bancha makes an excellent breakfast or after-dinner beverage.

Barley, Pearl. A particular strain of barley native to China, pearl barley grows easily in colder climates. It is good in stews and mixed with other grains such as rice. It is effective in breaking down animal fats in the body.

Black Sesame Seeds. Small black seeds, occasionally used as a garnish or in black *gomashio*, a condiment. A different variety of seed from the common tan sesame seed.

Brown Rice. Whole, unpolished rice. It is available in three varieties: short, medium, and long-grain, and contains an ideal balance of minerals, protein, and carbohydrates.

Burdock. A hardy plant that grows wild throughout the U.S. The long, dark burdock root is delicious in soups, stews, and sea-vegetable dishes,

*Italicized words are defined in glossary.

or sautéed with carrots. It is highly valued in macrobiotic cooking for its strengthening qualities.

Chemical Additives. Any of the various artificial flavorings, coloring agents, or preservatives, not naturally found in foods, that are used in refining and processing. Over three thousand chemical additives have been approved by the U.S. Food and Drug Administration.

Chinese Cabbage. A large, leafy vegetable with pale green tops and thick white stems. Sometimes called nappa, this juicy, slightly sweet vegetable is good in soups and stews, vegetable dishes, and pickled.

Cholesterol. A compound manufactured in the human body, important in the structure of membranes and the formation of certain hormones. Cholesterol is also a constituent of all animal products. Medical studies point to a relationship between excess consumption of cholesterol and the incidence of cancer.

Complex Carbohydrates. Those starches, known chemically as polysaccharides, that provide the body with a high proportion of usable energy over a period of several hours. Complex carbohydrates are the major components of the macrobiotic diet. A source of energy, they are supplied primarily by whole grains, vegetables, and beans.

Daikon. A long, white radish. Besides making a delicious side dish, daikon is a specific aid in dissolving fat and *mucus* deposits that have accumulated as a result of past animal food intake. Grated daikon aids in the digestion of oily foods.

Dried Daikon. Many natural food stores now carry packaged daikon that has been shredded and dried. This is especially good cooked with *kombu* and seasoned with a little *tamari*. Soaking dried daikon before use brings out its natural sweetness.

Dried Tofu. Tofu that has been naturally dehydrated by freezing. Used in soups, stews, vegetable, and sea-vegetable dishes. Less fatty than regular tofu. See *Tofu*.

Dulse. A reddish-purple sea-vegetable used in soups, salads, and vegetable dishes. Very high in protein, Vitamin A, iodine, and phosphorous. Used for centuries in European cooking, dulse is now harvested on both sides of the North Atlantic (including off the coasts of Maine and Massachusetts).

Fiber. The indigestible portion of whole foods; particularly, the bran of whole grains and the outer skin of legumes, vegetables, and fruits. Fiber facilitates the passage of waste through the intestines. Foods that are refined, processed, or peeled are low in fiber. Medical studies point to a positive relationship between fiber consumption and low incidence of cancer of the colon.

Fu. A dried wheat *gluten* product. Available in thin sheets or thick round cakes. Used in soups, stews, and vegetable dishes. High in protein.

Ginger. A spicy, pungent, golden-colored root, used as a garnish or seasoning in cooking. Also used in such remedies as the ginger compress.

Gluten (Wheat). The sticky substance that remains after the bran has been kneaded and rinsed from whole wheat flour. Used to make *seitan* and *fu*.

Gomashio. A condiment made from roasted, ground sesame seeds and *sea salt*. Gomashio is a rich source of minerals and whole oil and can be sprinkled lightly on rice and other grains.

Goma Dulse Powder. A condiment made from ground, baked *dulse* and sesame seeds. Also rich in minerals and other essential nutrients. Used on hot cereals.

Green Nori Flakes. A sea-vegetable condiment made from a certain type of *nori*, different from the packaged variety. The flakes are rich in iron, calcium, and Vitamin A. Can be sprinkled on whole grains, vegetables, salads, and other dishes.

Hijiki. A dark brown sea-vegetable that turns black when dried. It has a wiry consistency, may be strong-tasting, and is high in calcium and protein. Hijiki imported from Japan or havested off the coast of Maine is available dried and packaged in most natural food stores.

Hokkaido Pumpkin. There are two varieties of Hokkaido pumpkin. One has a deep orange color and the other has a light green skin similar to Hubbard squash. Hokkaido pumpkins are available at many natural food stores and by mail order. They have a tough outer skin and are very sweet inside.

Japanese Black Soybeans. A special type of soybean grown in Japan. It may be used medicinally to treat female reproductive problems. In cooking, black beans are used in soups and side dishes.

Kinpira. A sautéed *burdock* or burdock-and-carrot dish that is seasoned with *tamari*. This hearty root vegetable dish imparts strength and vitality.

Kombu. A wide, thick, dark green sea-vegetable that grows in deep ocean water. Often cooked with vegetables and beans; and used in making condiments, candy, and soup stocks. A single strip of kombu may be re-used several times to flavor soups. Kombu is rich in essential minerals. Medical studies have reported kombu's effectiveness in helping to prevent a variety of cancers.

Kuzu. A white starch made from the root of the wild kuzu plant. In the U.S., the plant is often called kudzu. Used in making soups, sauces, gravies, desserts, and for medicinal purposes.

Lotus Root. The root and seeds of a water lily which is brown-skinned with a hollow, chambered, off-white inside. Especially good for the respiratory organs. The seeds are used in grain, bean, and sea-vegetable dishes.

Macrobiotics. An approach to balanced living, based on a balanced diet, moderate exercise, harmony with the environment, and an understanding of the philosophic principles of *yin* and *yang*. George Ohsawa was the first to recognize how these traditional concepts could be applied to modern living.

Millet.   This small, yellow grain, which comes in many varieties, can be eaten on a regular basis. It can be used in soups or vegetable dishes, or eaten as a cereal.

Mirin.   A wine made from whole grain sweet rice. Used occasionally as a seasoning in vegetable or sea-vegetable dishes.

Miso.   A fermented grain or bean paste made from ingredients such as soybeans, barley, and rice. There are many varieties of miso now available. Barley (mugi) or soybean (hatcho) miso is usually recommended for daily use. Miso is especially good for the the circulatory and digestive organs. It is high in protein and Vitamin B_{12}.

Miso, Puréed.   Miso that has been reduced to a texture that will allow it to blend easily with other ingredients. To purée miso, place it in a bowl or *suribachi* and add enough water or broth to make a smooth paste. Blend with a wooden pestle or spoon.

Mochi.   A rice cake or dumpling made from cooked, pounded sweet rice.

Mucus.   Secretion of mucous membranes, normally serving to protect and lubricate main parts of the body. Illness, environmental pollution, smoking, and the consumption of excess fats, sugar, and flour products can stimulate the overproduction of *mucus* and clog body passageways, preventing the body from expelling harmful substances.

Nishime.   A method of cooking in which different combinations of vegetables, sea-vegetables, or soybean products are cut in large pieces and simmered for a long time over a low flame. Nishime is seasoned with *tamari* or *miso*, and cooked until almost all the water in the pot is gone. The ingredients become soft, sweet, and easily digested. Also referred to as waterless cooking.

Nori.   Thin sheets of dried sea-vegetable that are black or dark purple when dried. Nori is often roasted over a flame until green. It is used as a garnish, wrapped around *rice balls* in making *sushi*, or cooked with *tamari* as a condiment. Rich in Vitamin A and protein, nori also contains calcium, iron, Vitamins B_1, B_2, C, and D.

Ohitashi.   A method of boiling for leafy green vegetables sliced or whole. Water is boiled, vegetables are added and boiled from several seconds to a minute. Sometimes referred to as blanching.

Organic Foods.   Foods grown and harvested without the use of synthetically-compounded chemical fertilizers, pesticides, herbicides, and fungicides.

Polyunsaturated Fats.   Term used to describe the molecular structure of the fats that are present in vegetable oils and other whole foods, including fish. While polyunsaturates are more healthful than saturated fats, overconsumption may lead to elevated fatty acid (triglyceride) levels in the bloodstream.

Pressed Salad. Very thinly sliced or shredded fresh vegetables, combined with a pickling agent such as *sea salt*, *umeboshi*, grain vinegar, or *tamari*, and placed in a special pickle press. In the pickling process, many of the enzymes and vitamins are retained while the vegetables become easier to digest.

Preventive Diet. A diet whose goal is to reduce the risks of contracting a disease. Preventive diets exclude foods that have been linked to the formation of a disease and include foods that have been linked to the prevention of that disease.

Rice Balls. Rice shaped into balls or triangles, usually with a piece of *umeboshi* in the center, and wrapped in toasted *nori* or *shiso* leaves to completely cover. Pickles, seeds, vegetables, fried *tofu*, and other ingredients can be placed in the center to create a variety of tastes. Rice balls can also be coated with whole or ground sesame seeds.

Saturated Fats. Term used to describe the molecular structure of most of the fats found in red meats, dairy products, and other animal foods. Medical studies have linked the overconsumption of animal fats to the incidence of cancer.

Sea Salt. Salt obtained from evaporated sea water, as opposed to rock salt. It is either sun-baked or kiln-baked. High in trace minerals, it contains no harmful chemicals, sugar, or iodine.

Seitan. Wheat gluten cooked in *tamari*, *kombu*, and water. Seitan can be made at home or purchased ready-made at many natural food stores. Many people use it as a meat substitute.

Sesame Butter. A nut butter obtained by roasting and grinding sesame seeds until smooth and creamy. Used like peanut butter or in salad dressings and sauces.

Shiitake Mushrooms. Dried shiitake are imported from Japan. Fresh shiitake, grown in the U.S., have recently come on the market. Either type can be used in soup stocks or vegetable dishes, and dried shiitake are used in medicinal preparations. These mushrooms are effective in helping the body to discharge excess salt and animal fats.

Shio Kombu. Pieces of *kombu* cooked for a long time in *tamari* and used as a condiment. Use only a few pieces at a time, as shio kombu has a strong, salty taste.

Shio Nori. Pieces of *nori* cooked for a long time in *tamari* and water. Used occasionally as a condiment, shio nori is particularly tasty as a relish.

Shiso. A red, pickled leaf. The plant is known in English as the beefsteak plant. It is used to color *umeboshi* plums and as a condiment. Sometimes called chiso.

Simple Sugars. A source of quick, but short-lasting, energy. Simple sugars include sucrose (table sugar), fructose, glucose (dextrose), and lactose (milk sugar). Up to fifty percent of the carbohydrates consumed in the average modern diet are simple sugars.

Suribachi.   A special, serrated, glazed clay bowl. Used with a pestle, called a surikogi, for grinding and puréeing foods. An essential item in a macrobiotic kitchen, the suribachi can be used in a variety of ways to make condiments, spreads, dressings, baby foods, nut butters, and medicinal preparations.

Surikogi.   A wooden pestle that is used with a *suribachi*. Used to make *gomashio*, sea-vegetable powders, and other condiments, and to mash foods to obtain a creamy consistency.

Sushi.   Rice rolled with vegetables, fish, or pickles, wrapped in *nori*, and sliced in rounds. Sushi is becoming increasingly popular throughout the U.S. The best-quality macrobiotic sushi is made with brown rice and other natural ingredients.

Sushi Mat.   Very thin strips of bamboo that are fastened together with cotton thread so that they can be rolled tightly yet allow air to pass through freely. Used in rolling sushi, and also to cover freshly-cooked foods or leftovers.

Sweet Brown Rice.   A sweeter-tasting, more glutinous variety of rice. Used in *mochi*, ohagi, dumplings, and other dishes, it is often used in cooking for festive occasions.

Tamari.   Name given by George Ohsawa to traditional, naturally made soy sauce to distinguish it from commercial, chemically processed varieties. Original tamari is the liquid poured off during the process of making hatcho *miso*. The best quality tamari soy sauce is naturally fermented over two summers and is made from round soybeans and *sea salt* that is not highly refined.

Taro.   A type of potato with a thick, dark brown, hairy skin. Used as a vegetable or in the preparation of plasters for medicinal purposes. Also called albi.

Tekka.   A condiment made from hatcho *miso*, sesame oil, *burdock*, *lotus root*, carrot, and *ginger* root, sautéed on a low flame for several hours.

Tempeh.   A dish made from split soybeans, water, and a special bacteria, that is allowed to ferment for several hours. Tempeh is eaten in Indonesia and Sri Lanka as a staple food. It is available prepacked, ready to prepare, in some natural food stores. Rich in Vitamin B_{12} and protein.

Tofu.   Soybean curd, made from soybeans and nigari (a coagulant taken from salt water). Used in soups, vegetable dishes, dressings, etc., tofu is high in protein and does not contain animal fats. See *Dried Tofu*.

Udon.   Japanese noodles made from wheat, whole wheat, or whole wheat and unbleached white flour. Udon generally have a lighter flavor than soba (buckwheat) noodles.

Umeboshi.   Salty, pickled plums. Umeboshi plums stimulate the appetite and digestion and aid in maintaining an alkaline blood quality. *Shiso* leaves are usually added to the plums during pickling to impart a reddish color and natural flavoring.

Umeboshio Vinegar.   A salty, sour vinegar made from umeboshi plums. Diluted with water and used in sweet and sour sauces, salads, salad dressings, etc.

Unsaturated Fats.   See *Polyunsaturated Fats*.

Wakame.   A long, thin, green sea-vegetable used in making soups, salads, and vegetable dishes. High in protein, iron, and magnesium, wakame has a sweet taste and delicate texture and is especially good in *miso* soup.

Wheat Berries.   The grains of whole wheat are often called wheat berries. Wheat berries are good when soaked and pressure-cooked together with brown rice.

Wild Rice.   A wild grass that grows in water and is harvested by hand. Eaten traditionally by native Americans in Minnesota and other areas.

Yang.   In macrobiotics, energy or movement that has a centripetal or inward direction. One of the two antagonistic, yet complementary, forces that together describe all phenomena, yang is traditionally symbolized by a triangle (△).

Yin.   In macrobiotics, energy or movement that has a centrifugal or outward direction and results in expansion. One of the two antagonistic, yet complementary, forces that together describe all phenomena, yin is traditionally symbolized by an inverted triangle (▽).

Resources

MACROBIOTIC WAY OF LIFE SEMINAR

The Macrobiotic Way of Life Seminar is an introductory program offered by the Kushi Institute in Boston. It includes classes in macrobiotic cooking, home care, kitchen setup, lectures on the philosophy of macrobiotics and the standard diet, and individual way of life guidance. It is presented monthly and includes introductory and intermediate level programs. Information on the Way of Life Seminar is available from:

> The Kushi Institute
> 17 Station Street
> Brookline, Massachusetts 02146
> (617) 738-0045

MACROBIOTIC RESIDENTIAL SEMINAR

The Macrobiotic Residential Seminar is an introductory program offered at the Kushi Foundation Berkshires Center in Becket, Massachusetts. It is a one week live-in program that includes hands-on training in macrobiotic cooking and home care, lectures on the philosophy and practice of macrobiotics, and meals prepared by a specially trained cooking staff. It is presented monthly and includes introductory and intermediate levels. Information on the Macrobiotic Residential Seminar is available from:

> Kushi Foundation Berkshires Center
> Box 7
> Becket, Massachusetts 01223
> (413) 623-5742

KUSHI INSTITUTE LEADERSHIP STUDIES

For those who wish to study further, the Kushi Institute offers instruction for individuals who wish to become trained and certified macrobiotic teachers. Leadership training programs are also offered at Kushi Institute affiliates in London, Amsterdam, Antwerp, Florence, as well as in Portugal and Switzerland. Information on Leadership Studies is available from the Kushi Institute in Boston, Massachusetts.

OTHER PROGRAMS

The Kushi Institute offers a variety of public programs including an annual Summer Conference in western Massachusetts, special weight-loss and natural beauty seminars, and intensive cooking and spiritual development training at the Berkshires Center. Moreover, a variety of introductory and public programs are offered through an international network of over 300 educational centers in the United States, Canada, and throughout the world. The Kushi Foundation publishes a *Worldwide Macrobiotic Directory* every year listing these centers and individuals. Please consult the *Directory* for the nearest macrobiotic center or qualified instructor.

PUBLICATIONS

Michio and Aveline Kushi have authored numerous books on macrobiotic cooking, philosophy, diet, and way of life. These titles are listed in the Recommended Reading list and are available at macrobiotic centers, natural food stores, and bookstores. Ongoing developments are reported in the *East West Journal,* a monthly magazine begun in 1971 with an international readership of 200,000. The *Journal* features regular articles on the macrobiotic approach to health and nutrition, as well as related subjects. It is available at most natural food stores and by subscription.

Recommended Reading

Aihara, Cornellia. *The Dō of Cooking*. Chico, Calif.: George Ohsawa Macrobiotic Foundation, 1972.

_____. *Macrobiotic Childcare*. Oroville, Calif.: George Ohsawa Macrobiotic Foundation, 1971.

Aihara, Herman. *Basic Macrobiotics*. Tokyo & New York: Japan Publications, Inc., 1985.

Benedict, Dirk. *Confessions of a Kamikaze Cowboy*. Garden City Park, N.Y.: Avery Publishing Group, 1991.

Brown, Virginia, with Susan Stayman. *Macrobiotic Miracle: How A Vermont Family Overcame Cancer*. Tokyo & New York: Japan Publications, Inc., 1985.

Dietary Goals for the United States. Washington, D. C.: Select Committee on Nutrition and Human Needs, U.S. Senate, 1977.

Diet, Nutrition and Cancer. Washington, D. C.: National Academy of Sciences, 1982.

Dufty, William. *Sugar Blues*. New York: Warner Books, 1975.

Esko, Edward and Wendy Esko. *Macrobiotic Cooking for Everyone*. Tokyo & New York: Japan Publications, Inc., 1980.

Esko, Wendy. *Aveline Kushi's Introducing Macrobiotic Cooking*. Tokyo and New York: Japan Publications, Inc., 1987.

Fukuoka, Masanobu. *The Natural Way of Farming*. Tokyo & New York: Japan Publications, Inc., 1985.

_____. *The One-Straw Revolution*. Emmaus, Pa.: Rodale Press, 1978.

Healthy People: The Surgeon General's Report on Health Promotion and Disease Prevention. Washington, D. C.: Government Printing Office, 1979.

Hiedenry, Carolyn. *Making the Transition to a Macrobiotic Diet*. Garden City Park, N.Y.: Avery Publishing Group, 1987.

Hippocrates. *Hippocratic Writings*. Edited by G. E. R. Lloyd. Translated by J. Chadwick and W. N. Mann. New York: Penguin Books, 1978.

I Ching or *Book of Changes*. Translated by Richard Wilhelm and Cary F. Baynes. Princeton: Bollingen Foundation, 1950.

Ineson, John. *The Way of Life: Macrobiotics and the Spirit of Christianity*. Tokyo & New York: Japan Publications, Inc., 1986.

Jacobs, Leonard and Barbara Leonard. *Cooking with Seitan*. Tokyo & New York: Japan Publications, Inc., 1986.

Jacobson, Michael. *The Changing American Diet*. Washington, D. C.: Center for Science in the Public Interest, 1978.

Kaibara, Ekiken. *Yojokun: Japanese Secrets of Good Health*. Tokyo: Tokuma Shoten, 1974.

Kidder, Ralph D. and Edward F. Kelley. *Choice for Survival: The Baby Boomer's Dilemma*. Tokyo & New York: Japan Publications, Inc., 1987.

Kohler, Jean and Mary Alice. *Healing Miracles from Macrobiotics*. West Nyack, N. Y.: Parker, 1979.

Kotsch, Ronald. *Macrobiotics: Yesterday and Today*. Tokyo & New York: Japan Publications, Inc., 1985.

Kushi, Aveline. *How to Cook with Miso*. Tokyo & New York: Japan Publications, Inc., 1978.

_____. *Lessons of Night and Day*. Garden City Park, N.Y.: Avery Publishing Group, 1985.

_____. *Macrobiotic Food and Cooking Series: Diabetes and Hypoglycemia; Allergies*. Tokyo & New York: Japan Publications, Inc., 1985.

_____. *Macrobiotic Food and Cooking Series: Obesity, Weight Loss, and Eating Disorders; Infertility and Reproductive Disorders*. Tokyo & New York: Japan Publications, Inc., 1987.

Kushi, Aveline, with Alex Jack. *Aveline Kushi's Complete Guide to Macrobiotic Cooking*. New York: Warner Books, 1985.

Kushi, Aveline and Michio Kushi. *Macrobiotic Pregnancy and Care of the Newborn*. Edited by Edward and Wendy Esko. Tokyo & New York: Japan Publications, Inc., 1984.

_____. *Macrobiotic Child Care and Family Health*. Tokyo & New York: Japan Publications, Inc., 1986.

Kushi, Aveline, and Wendy Esko. *Macrobiotic Family Favorites*. Tokyo & New York: Japan Publications, Inc., 1987.

Kushi, Aveline, and Wendy Esko. *The Changing Seasons Macrobiotic Cookbook*. Garden City Park, N.Y.: Avery Publishing Group, 1983.

Kushi, Michio. *The Book of Dō-In: Exercise for Physical and Spiritual Development*. Tokyo & New York: Japan Publications, Inc. 1979.

_____. *The Book of Macrobiotics: The Universal Way of Health, Happiness and Peace*. Tokyo & New York: Japan Publications, Inc., 1986 (Rev. ed.).

_____. *Cancer and Heart Disease: The Macrobiotic Approach to Degenerative Disorders*. Tokyo & New York: Japan Publications, Inc., 1986 (Rev. ed.).

_____. *Crime and Diet: The Macrobiotic Approach*. Tokyo & New York: Japan Publications, Inc., 1987.

_____. *The Era of Humanity*. Brookline, Mass.: East West Journal, 1980.

_____. *How to See Your Health: The Book of Oriental Diagnosis*. Tokyo & New York: Japan Publications, Inc., 1980.

_____. *Macrobiotic Health Education Series: Diabetes and Hypoglycemia; Allergies*. Tokyo & New York: Japan Publications, Inc., 1985.

_____. *Macrobiotic Health Education Series: Obesity, Weight Loss, and Eating Disorders; Infertility and Reproductive Disorders*. Tokyo & New York: Japan Publications, Inc., 1987.

_____. *Natural Healing through Macrobiotics*. Tokyo & New York: Japan Publications, Inc., 1978.

_____. *On the Greater View: Collected Thoughts on Macrobiotics and Humanity*. Garden City Park, N.Y.: Avery Publishing Group, 1985.

_____. *Your Face Never Lies*. Garden City Park, N.Y.: Avery Publishing Group, 1983.

Kushi, Michio, and Alex Jack. *The Cancer Prevention Diet*. New York: St. Martin's Press, 1983.

_____. *Diet for a Strong Heart*. New York: St. Martin's Press, 1984.

Kushi, Michio, with Alex Jack. *One Peaceful World*. New York: St. Martin's Press, 1987.

Kushi, Michio, with Edward and Wendy Esko. *Gentle Art of Making Love, The*. Garden City Park, N.Y.: Avery Publishing Group, 1990.

Kushi, Michio and Aveline Kushi, with Alex Jack. *The Macrobiotic Diet*. Tokyo & New York: Japan Publications, Inc., 1985.

Kushi, Michio, and the East West Foundation. *The Macrobiotic Approach to Cancer*. Garden City Park, N.Y.: Avery Publishing Group, 1982.

Kushi, Michio, with Stephen Blauer. *The Macrobiotic Way*. Garden City Park, N.Y.: Avery Publishing Group, 1985.

Lerman, Andrea Bliss. *Macrobiotic Community Cookbook, The*. Garden City Park, N.Y.: Avery Publishing Group, 1989.

Mendelsohn, Robert S., M.D. *Confessions of a Medical Heretic*. Chicago: Contemporary Books, 1979.

_____. *Male Practice*. Chicago: Contemporary Books, 1980.

Nussbaum, Elaine. *Recovery: From Cancer to Health through Macrobiotics*. Tokyo & New York: Japan Publications, Inc., 1986.

Nutrition and Mental Health. Washington, D. C.: Select Committee on Nutrition and Human Needs, U.S. Senate, 1977, 1980.

Ohsawa, George. *Cancer and the Philosophy of the Far East*. Oroville, Calif.: George Ohsawa Macrobiotic Foundation, 1971 edition.

_____. *You Are All Sanpaku*. Edited by William Dufty. New York: University Books, 1965.

_____. *Zen Macrobiotics*. Los Angeles: Ohsawa Foundation, 1965.

Price, Western, A., D. D. S. *Nutrition and Physical Degeneration*. Santa Monica, Calif.: Price-Pottenger Nutritional Foundation, 1945.

Sattilaro, Anthony, M. D., with Tom Monte. *Recalled by Life: The Story of My Recovery from Cancer.* Boston: Houghton-Mifflin, 1982.

Schauss, Alexander. *Diet, Crime, and Delinquency.* Berkeley, Calif.: Parker House, 1980.

Scott, Neil E., with Jean Farmer. *Eating with Angels.* Tokyo & New York: Japan Publications, Inc., 1986.

Tara, William. *A Challenge to Medicine.* Tokyo & New York: Japan Publications, Inc., 1987.

_____. *Macrobiotics and Human Behavior.* Tokyo & New York: Japan Publications, Inc., 1985.

Yamamoto, Shizuko. *Barefoot Shiatsu.* Tokyo & New York: Japan Publications, Inc., 1979.

The Yellow Emperor's Classic of Internal Medicine. Translated by Ilza Veith, Berkeley: University of California Press, 1949.

Index

Other titles of interest

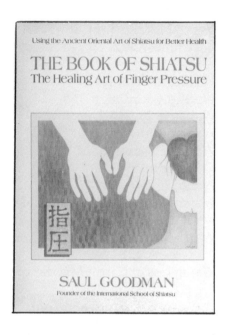

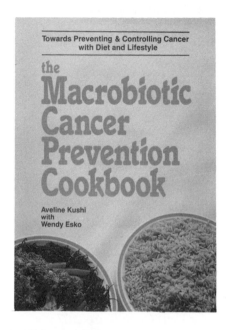

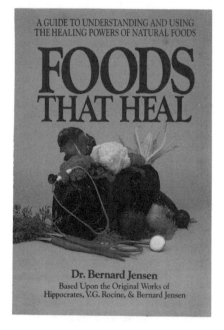

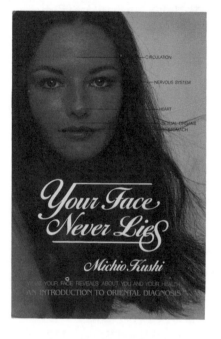

Ask for these titles at your local bookstore or health food shop.
For a complete Avery catalog, call us toll-free at 1-800-548-5757.

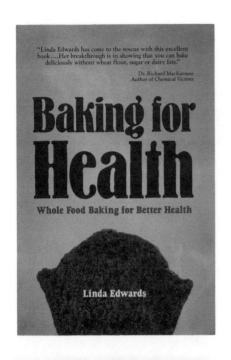

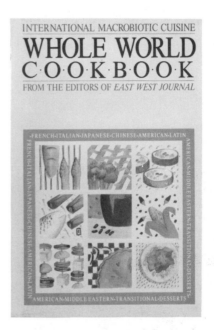

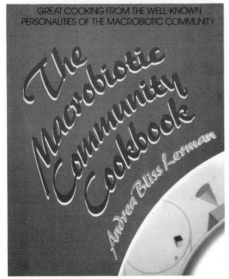

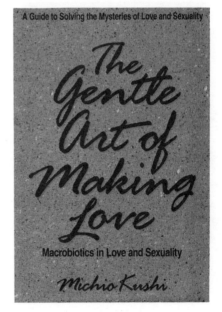

Ask for these titles at your local bookstore or health food shop.
For a complete Avery catalog, call us toll-free at 1-800-548-5757.

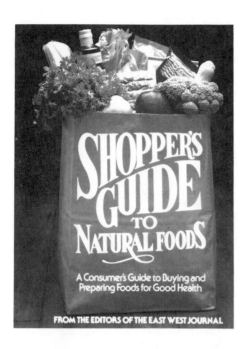

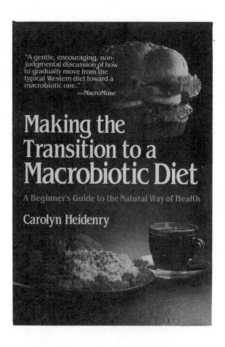

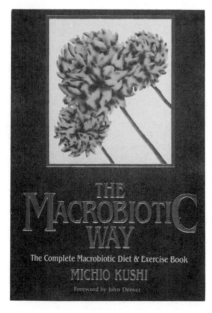

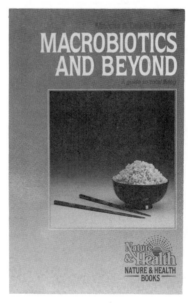

Ask for these titles at your local bookstore or health food shop.
For a complete Avery catalog, call us toll-free at 1-800-548-5757.

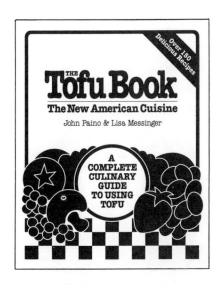

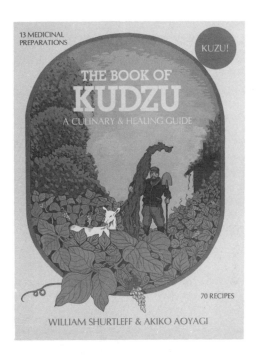

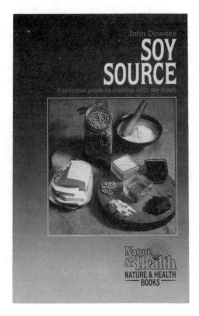

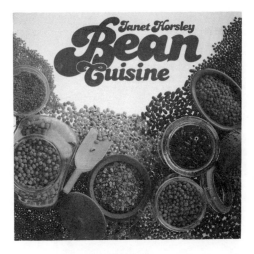

Ask for these titles at your local bookstore or health food shop.
For a complete Avery catalog, call us toll-free at 1-800-548-5757.

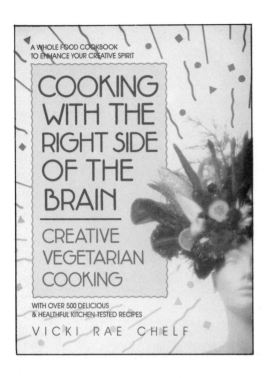
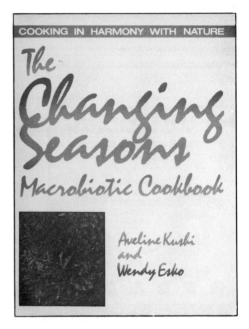
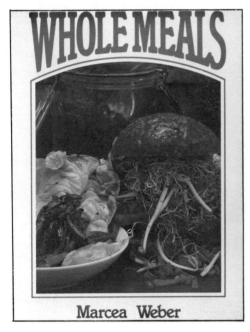
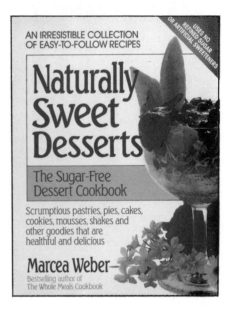